ANCIENT EGYPTIAN ECONOMICS
The Timeless Philosophy
Of
Physical, Mental and Spiritual Wealth

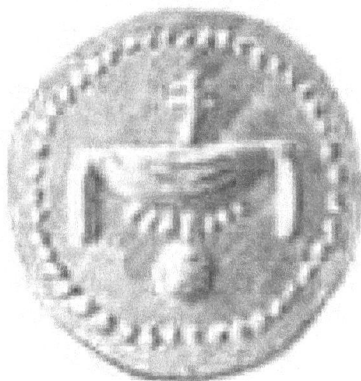

By
Sebai Dr. Muata Ashby

Ancient Egyptian Economics

Sema Institute/Cruzian Mystic Books
P.O. Box 570459
Miami, Florida, 33257
(305) 378-6253 Fax: (305) 378-6253

First U.S. edition © 2011 By Reginald Muata Ashby

The author is available for group lectures and individual counseling. For further information contact the publisher.

Ashby, Muata
ANCIENT EGYPTIAN ECONOMICS
Kemetic Wisdom of Saving and Investing in Wealth of Body, Mind, and Soul for Building True Civilization, Prosperity and Spiritual Enlightenment
ISBN: 1-884564-13-5

Library of Congress Cataloging in Publication Data

Other books by Muata Ashby

See catalog in the back section for more listings

2

TABLE OF CONTENTS

TABLE OF FIGURES

Foreword

Question: Why has the subject of finances and economics become important, I thought the spiritual teachings and Ancient Egyptian Philosophy and money were separate?

Answer:

Finances and money are an integral part of Ancient Egyptian culture as an instrument for promoting Maat ethics in the form of the well-being of the '*hekat*'. The hekat are the people and the "*Heka*" is the Pharaoh. The Pharaoh was like a shepherd leading a flock and moneys were controlled righteously to promote the welfare of the people. In that tradition we have applied the philosophy of maatian economics to promote the well-being of those who are following this path as well as those who may read the books so they may avoid financial trouble as much as possible and have better capacity to practice the teachings. In order to have a successful life, human beings need a certain amount of money and wealth, but money and wealth are not the goal. They are a foundation that enables the true goal of life, enlightenment, to be realized. Therefore, we are only fulfilling the duty of transmitting wisdom about wealth to promote maat,righteousness, truth and well-being, for all. This volume explores the mysteries of wealth based on the teachings of the sages of Ancient Egypt and the means to promote prosperity that allows a person to create the conditions for discovering inner peace and spiritual enlightenment.
HTP-Peace

PART 1:
Introduction to Kemetic "Ancient Egyptian" Economics

Misuse of Ancient Egyptian Symbols in Western Iconography

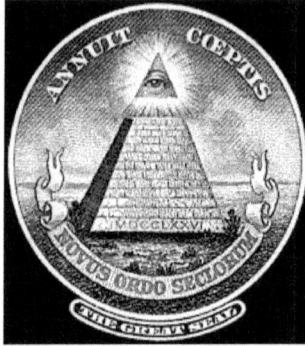

Figure 1: Pyramid and All seeing Eye on the US Dollar Bill

Why are Ancient Egyptian Symbols used by the United States of America Government and what does it mean?

Before going deeply into the history and philosophy of Ancient Egyptian economics, we will work backwards from the present day use of Ancient Egyptian symbols to their origins in Ancient Egypt. Before going forward it is important to understand that when we speak of Ancient Egypt, we are referring to the culture and wisdom of the people who lived in the land today called Egypt, but before the arrival of the Greeks, Romans, Christians and Muslims. In that period (5000 B.C.E. to 300 B.C.E.), the inhabitants referred to the land by the name of "Kemet" –"the black land." This is where we get the term "Kemetic Economics" from.

8

Many symbols of Ancient Egypt (ancient name: Kamit or Kemet) appear in architecture, literature, and other iconography of the U.S.A. Why is this, and what is it supposed to mean? Many people know that several of the "founding Fathers"[1] of the U.S.A. were "freemasons". Originally Freemasons were men in the British Empire who were part of guilds. In the context of influencing the condition of society, Freemasonry is a group of men forming a fraternal secret order, as in a cabal, to control the activities of government and society; in other words, they have secret alliances beyond those of open government. Many Ancient Egyptian symbols and architectural forms were adopted by practitioners of Freemasonry and some of the groups claim to have a lineage that goes back to Ancient Egypt, but that is impossible since the first freemason groups were known to have developed in Europe within the last millennium, a period well after the Ancient Egyptian. So it is important to understand that Ancient Kemetic (Ancient Egyptian) culture was, unlike the Masonic order, governed with a philosophy based on ethical culture to be applied to all citizens. That ethical culture, termed "Maat," was not only the foundation of the government and courts but also the foundation of the Ancient Egyptian temple system. In fact Maat is a philosophy, as well as a goddess of order, truth, righteousness and justice. In the last 500 years, western culture has been able to study and adopt many aspects of other cultures that they met and were influenced, by or which they conquered. Many things were co-opted and others were used without

---

[1] The signatories of the Declaration of Independence are often referred to as "Founders". George Washington was dominant person during this time.

9

their intrinsic original intent or meaning. When studying or following the culture, history and philosophy of Ancient Egypt, it is necessary to distinguish between what has been presented in modern times as Ancient Egyptian culture through modern day usage of Ancient Egyptian symbols by organizations which purport to follow the Ancient Egyptian teachings and may even claim to be descendants of the original teachers, as opposed to the actual history and teachings of Ancient Egypt.

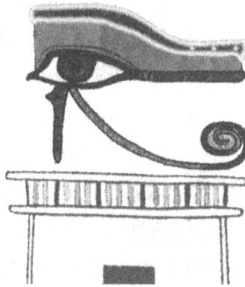

Figure 2: The Ancient Egyptian Eye of Spiritual Awakening

In the case of the U.S.A., many of the symbols were used without adopting the original meaning and intent. A primary example is the all-seeing eye on the U.S.A. Dollar Bill. It is important to understand that the Ancient Egyptian Mysteries (Shetaut Neter, as symbolized by the open eye) are not the same teachings followed by organizations which in modern times refer to themselves as *fraternal orders, lodges, masons, freemasons, illuminati, Odd Fellows, Shriners, new world orders, Satanists, occultists,* or *psychics.* In fact, the organizations just mentioned have their origins in Western countries and not in Ancient Africa (Kemet), although the iconographies of the original Grand Temples of the Mystery Systems of Ancient Egypt might have influenced them.

So observers should be careful when examining the use of Ancient Egyptian symbols by modern organizations. For example, the use of the pyramid on the reverse of the seal of the United States dollar would seem to mean that the founding fathers of the United States had the idea of invoking the principles of the Ancient Egyptian tradition in the founding of the new country (United States). It was explained by the occultist and reputed expert in Masonic lore, Manly Hall, that many of the U.S. founding fathers were masons and that they received assistance from masons in Europe to establish the United States for *"a peculiar and particular purpose known only to the initiated few."* However, historians have documented that an impetus behind the secession from England and Europe and the support of the "Founding Fathers" of the U.S.A. was for the purpose, by some Europeans, of undermining certain powerful interests in Europe and thereby gaining economic advantages and political power by acquiring new lands and resources. Hall said that the seal was the signature of the masons and that the unfinished pyramid symbolizes the task that the government has to accomplish. The eagle is a representation of the phoenix, which is the ancient Greek reinterpretation of the Ancient Egyptian (ancient African) Benu bird (symbol of the god Ra and rebirth).

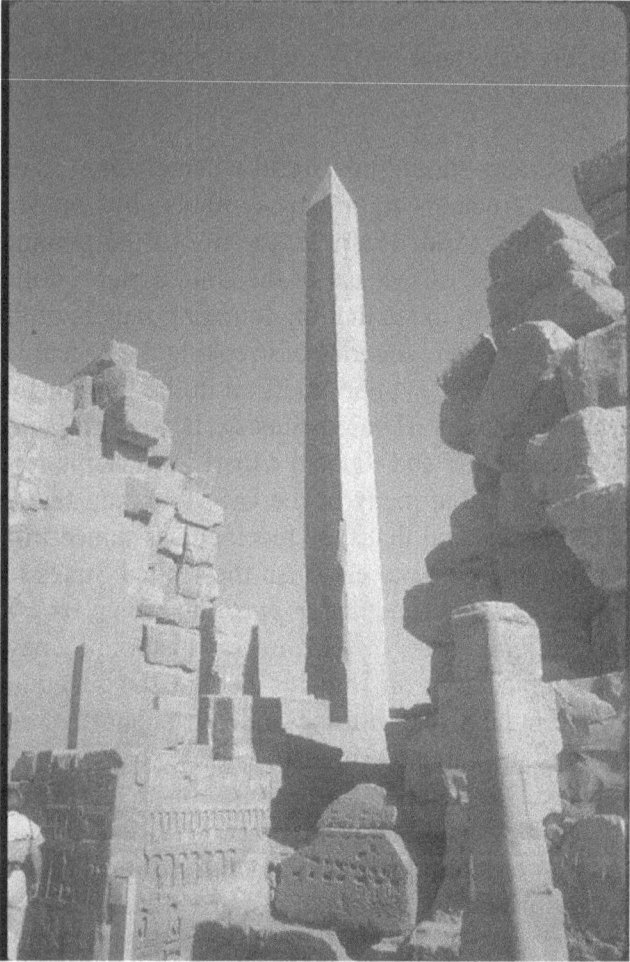

Figure 3: Above: Obelisk at Karnak Temple (Egypt)

While the Ancient Egyptian Obelisk is a monument to the God Geb and the Goddess Nut, the western obelisk is a monument to western culture.

Figure 4: Below: Washington Monument (replica of the
Ancient Egyptian obelisk)

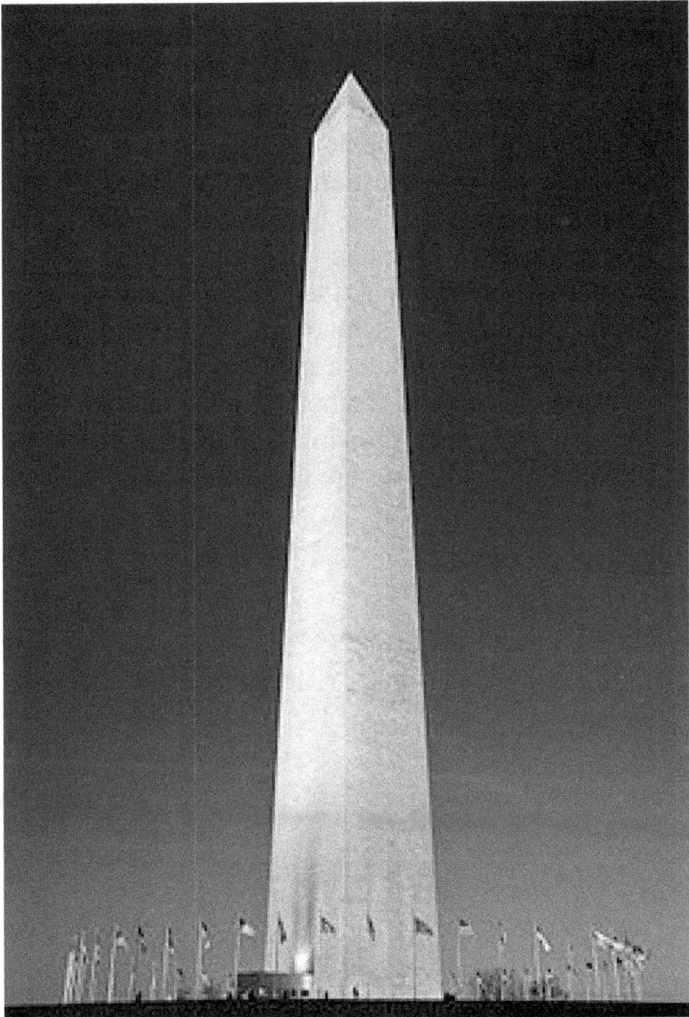

Another Ancient Egyptian symbol used to represent the United States is the Washington Monument, which is a copy of the Ancient Egyptian Obelisk. The Lincoln memorial and Mount Rushmore, two of the most important icons of the United States were admittedly (by their modern day creators) inspired by the Temple of Rameses II at Abu Simbel. So the question may be asked, if the founding fathers of the United States intended to use Ancient Egyptian representations, which essentially means that they are wishing to adopt their meaning and symbolism, why then did the founding fathers allow a government to be set up that is in almost complete contradiction with Ancient Egyptian principles? Some of the more obvious contradictions are listed below.

Figure 5: Below: Lincoln Memorial, using Ancient Kamitan (Egyptian) architecture for the posture of Lincoln.

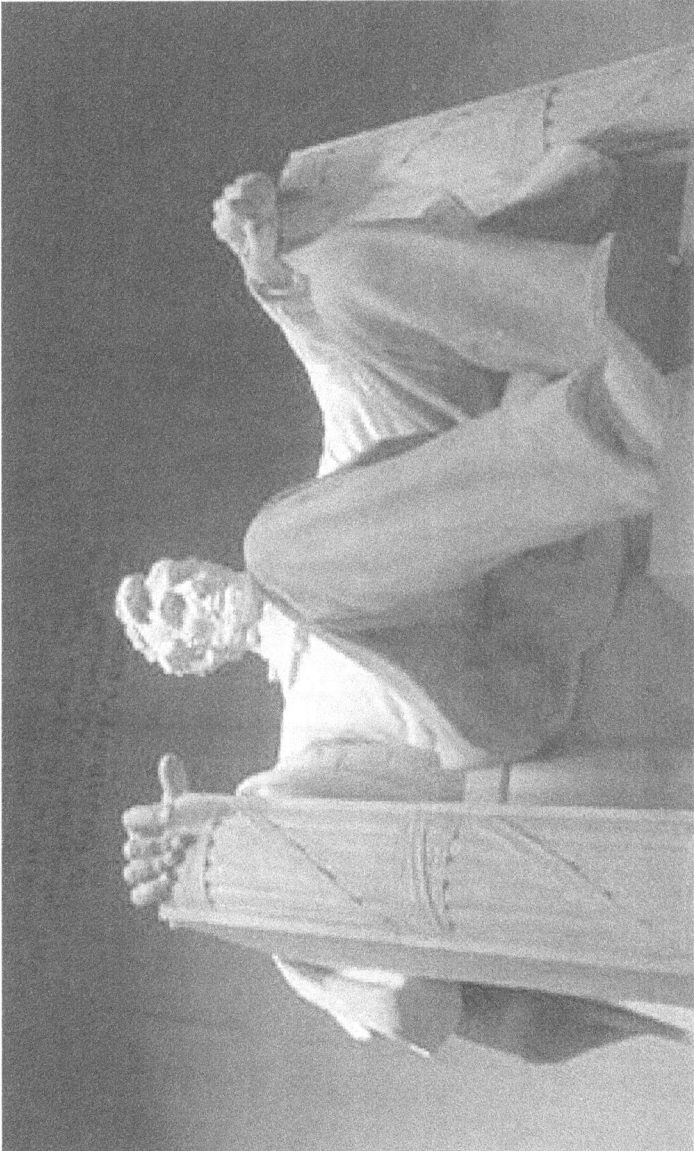

The Lincoln memorial and Mount Rushmore, two of the most important icons of the United States were admittedly inspired by the Massive Temple of Rameses II at Abu Simbel.

Figure 6: Below: Front of the Temple of Amun at Abu Simbel by Rameses the Great, dedicated to Amun-Ra and Ptah (c. 1279 B.C.E.)

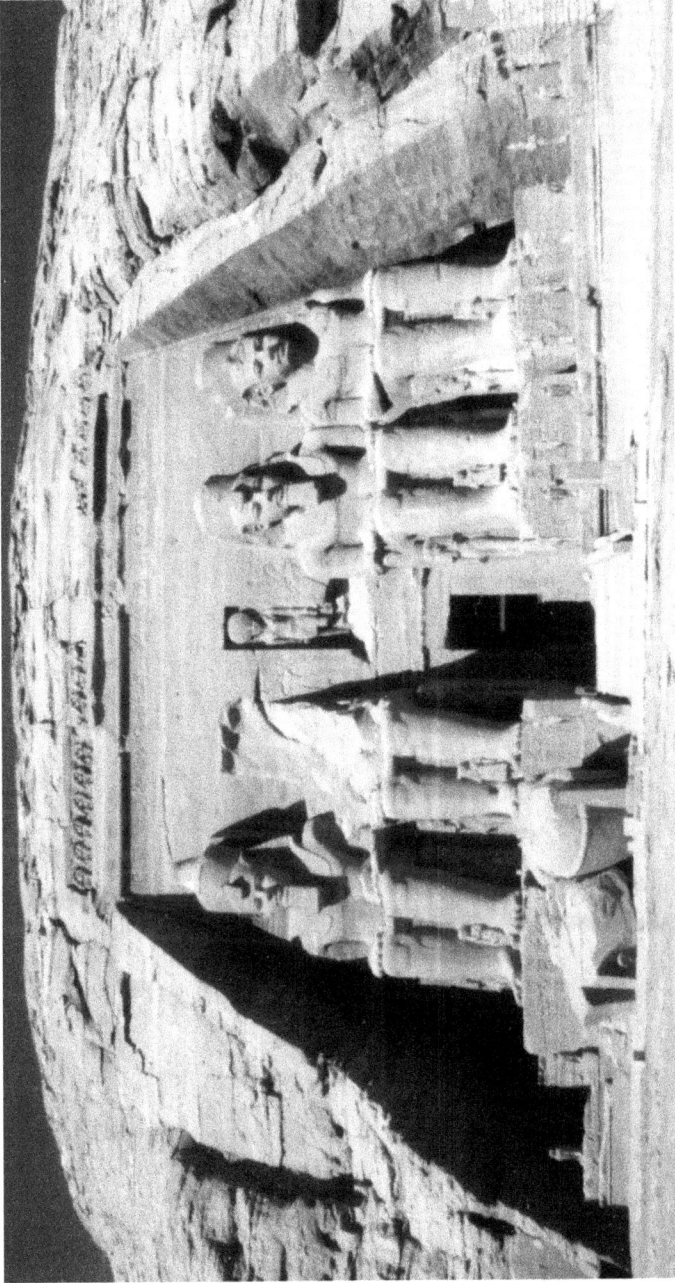

Figure 7: Mount Rushmore (United States of America)

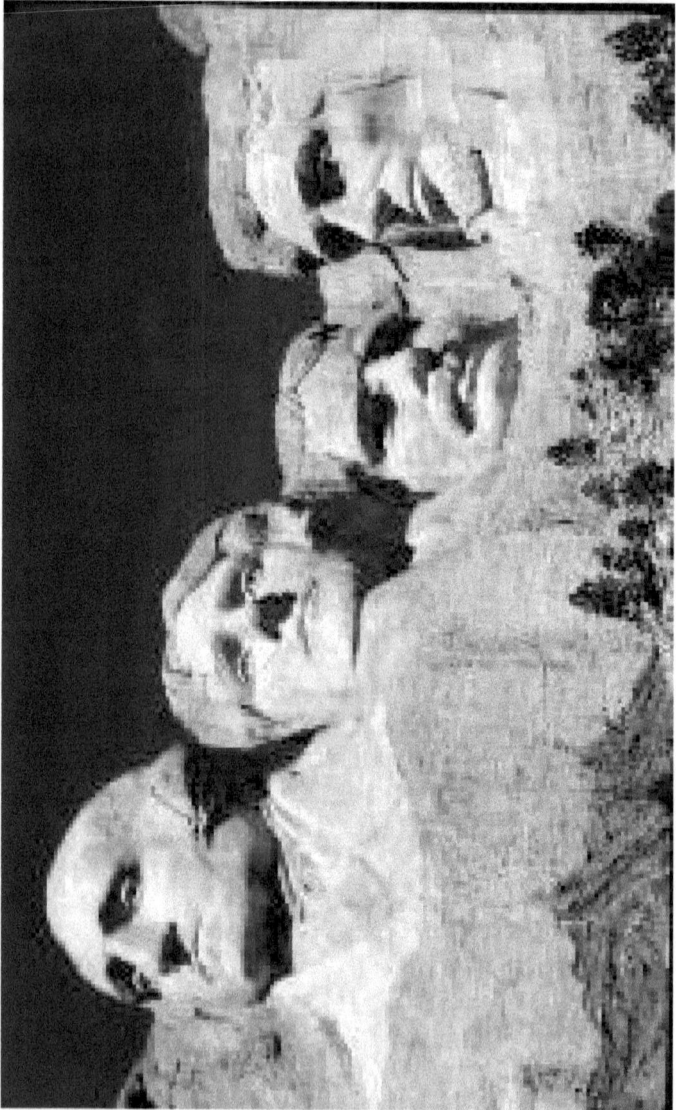

Ancient Egyptian Economics

Table 1: Differences between Ancient Egypt and the United States (Western Culture)

Ancient Egyptian Culture	Western (USA) Culture
1. In Ancient Egypt ,the equality of men and women was a standard.	1. In the United States women were relegated to the position of servitude to white men, with no voting rights. In the West women continue to be second class citizens, receiving lower pay than men and suffering other disparities.
2. Ancient Egypt did not engage in racism or racial slavery.	2. Modern western culture was founded on racism and racial slavery which dehumanizes people. In the United States, slavery was an economic boon and the country would not have developed into a superpower without it.
3. In Ancient Egypt religion was an integral part of the government and when a separation occurred, the degradation of culture and the downfall of society ensued.	3. The USA government system was based on a separation of government and church. In the United States there is a philosophy of separation of church and state which has led to corruption in government and business since the moral aspect of culture is actively

	detached from day to day life.
4. The initiatic principles of the pyramid related to a mystical spiritual awakening	4. The pyramid is used as a symbol of prestige and not as an initiatic symbol. Mysticism is actively shunned in the United States and other western countries though practiced in rudimentary forms by a few. The pyramid is seen as an architectural monument rather than a mystical symbol.
5. The obelisk is a tantric symbol relating to the union of the opposites in Creation – using sexual symbolism it represents the penis of the god Geb, who symbolizes earth and goddess Nut who symbolizes the Heavens. The union symbolizes a completeness of the soul with spirit. (Above and below).	5. The Washington monument is a symbol of the power of the government of the United States. The obelisk as a mystical tantric symbol in the United States is unknown. It is a symbol of power in the United States and therefore it is a projection of the lower sexual energy of western culture into technology, economics and politics to control the world, as opposed to a spiritual mystical goal.
6. The Temple of Abu Simbel contains	6. In the United States Mount Rushmore is a

monumental sculptures of the gods of Ancient Egypt, and therefore is a spiritual monument.	monumental sculpture dedicated to presidents, political leaders.
7. The Benu bird is the symbol of spiritual awakening and resurrection.	7. The Eagle is a symbol of political and military power.

The U.S.A. government took the Ancient Egyptian symbols of the Pyramid and the open eye to represent a supposed new world order based on the past order. However, the similarity between the Ancient Egyptian culture and the U.S.A. or Western culture ends there, and the disparity is evident in the misuse of religious symbols that has led to misunderstanding of the ancient tradition and misinformation about the present one. The study of Ancient Egyptian economics offers some insights into a workable form of economy that can demonstrate the vast differences between the economic systems and may also present solutions for current problems. Ancient Egyptian religion used the symbol of the spiritual eye[2] to represent the awakening of higher consciousness. There was recognition that in order for that awakening to occur, there needs to be virtue in a human being.

2 African Religion Vol 4: Asarian Theology by Muata Ashby

Fundamental Principles of Ancient Egyptian Economics

Gold was a storehouse of physical wealth but also seen as a reflection of timeless and immortal qualities of divinity, the sun, so possessing it represented closeness to the spiritual essence of the Divine.

-Muata Ashby

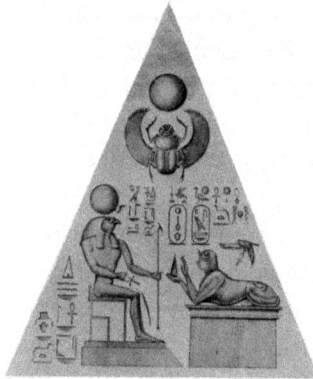

Figure 8: Ancient Egyptian BenBen Stone (Capstone)

The pinnacle of the obelisk is a reference to the Most High Spirit. In order to achieve that height, it is necessary to engage in a process of spiritual self-discovery which is based upon sound ethical conscience. According to Ancient Egyptian ethics (Maat philosophy), fundamental economics necessarily means non-stealing and proper distribution of wealth.

Ancient Egyptian Wisdom Teachings:

> "If thou be industrious to procure wealth, be generous in the disposal of it. One is never so happy as when giving happiness unto others."

> "An immoderate desire of riches is a poison lodged in the mind. It contaminates and destroys everything that was good in it. It is no sooner rooted there, than all virtue, all honesty, all natural affection, fly before the face of it."

> "O thou who are enamored with the beauties of Truth, and hast fixed thy heart on the simplicity of her charms, hold fast thy fidelity unto her, and forsake her not: the constancy of thy virtue shall crown thee with honor."

In order to have sustained prosperity, peace and security in a country, that country must be based on ethical principles. The Ancient Egyptians called that ethical principle "Maat." The Ancient Egyptian government is often referred to as a Theocracy, but a more accurate term would be "Ethiocracy" [Ethical-Theocracy]. Theocracy is a form of government based on religious law, but in Ancient Egypt, the government, as all other areas of society, was under the overall rubric of Maat Philosophy[3], the Ancient Egyptian theological, philosophical and ethical framework of spiritual, social, political and economic institutions. A theocratic form of government can be corrupted if the values followed are not based on virtue and morality, and if there is lacking commitment to truth and ethical conscience as opposed to moral relativism and political

---

[3] See the book Introduction to Maat Philosophy by Muata Ashby

expediency. The Christian Catholic Church suffered this problem of amoral government at various periods throughout its history, which led to social and religious decay, dissent, and the formation of the protestant movement. Moral theocracy is a kind of shepherding form of government. Morality here means that which is good, true, honest, compassionate, and fair, i.e. integrity, righteousness, justice, balance, peace, honor and honesty. Morality in the ancient sense cannot be equated with moral relativism or the novel concept of "new morality" or "alternative moral philosophy," which implies sexual freedom, or sexual revolution or situational morality. Maat implies universal moral/ethical principles that apply to all, but are not to be forced or imposed on other cultures or nations against their will. In Ancient Egypt, the laws had to be based on the philosophy of Maat. Maat is the concept of order, truth and balance in action, similar to Confucianism and Taoism of China, and Dharma of Buddhism. The following are injunctions of Maatian order contained in the teachings of the Ancient Egyptian Sage Amenemope.[4]

On Business and Commerce
Sage Amenemope
(48) Do not assess a man who has nothing,
And thus falsify your pen.
If you find a large debt against a poor man, Make it into three parts;
Forgive two, let one stand,
(49) You will find it a path of life.
(66) Haste not to be rich, but be not slothful in thine own interest.
(83) One does not run to reach success,

---

4 The 42 Precepts of Maat and the Philosophy of Righteous Action of the Wisdom Sages, by Muata Ashby (Ancient Egyptian Wisdom Texts)

One does not move to spoil it.
(108) Don't make yourself a ferry on the river, And
then strain to seek its fare;
(109) Take the fare from him who is wealthy,
And let pass him who is poor.

The 42 Precepts of Maat are condensed injunctions
that form the foundation of Maat Philosophy. They
are written in the form of negative statements ["I
have not.... Ex: Maat Precept: I have not snatched
away food from the needy] reflecting the successful
accomplishment of virtuous actions and refraining
from actions based on vice. However, in the
Ancient Egyptian wisdom texts, the Ancient
Egyptian sages expounded further on the practical
interpretation and application of the precepts in day-
to-day life.

> Do not move the scales, do not change the
> weights and do not diminish the parts of the
> bushel... Do not create a bushel that
> contains two, lest you will near the abyss.
> The bushel is the eye of Ra (God). He
> loathes him who defrauds.
>> The teachings of Sage Amenemope

The Ancient Egyptian culture and civilization was
the longest-lived and has the record as the longest
perpetual civilization [10,000 years][5] in human
history. One of the reasons for their success is that
the culture was founded and governed by an ethical
philosophy that discouraged and prevented
government excesses and economic frauds, unlike a
market economy or fiat currencies that promote
fraud, consumerism, boom and bust periods, over-
consumption and destruction of the environment.

---

5 see the book African Origins by Muata Ashby

(36) "I have never befouled the water." Variant: held back the water from flowing in its season. **(15) "I have not laid waste the ploughed lands."**
-Form Pert em Heru (Ancient Egyptian Book of Enlightenment)

The country was protected by a legal system that was based on the ethical philosophy of "Maat." Maat is a philosophy and a universal principle of cosmic order that all human beings need to observe in order to avoid strife and suffering and maintain personal balance, balance with the society, and balance with the universe and the Supreme Being (God). Therefore, any violation of Maat was a serious and egregious act that was dealt with forthwith so as to maintain the order of the society.[6]

"They who revere MAAT are long lived; they who are covetous have no tomb."
-Ancient Egyptian Proverb
-Sage Amenemope

Before the "Late Period," the Ancient Egyptians did not use coin money as modern society does today. When shopping in an Ancient Egyptian market people, would need to bargain on a price. There were few fixed prices, and Ancient Egyptians were experienced at calculating the cost of an item. Cost was measured in a unit called *deben*[7] which was a copper weight of .5 ounces.

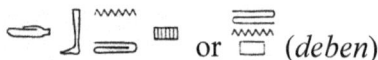

$$\text{or} \quad (deben)$$

---

6 see the book Introduction to Maat Philosophy by Muata Ashby
7 deben: about 92 grammes, ten kit equalled one deben.

The deben was a measure of weight used for silver and gold, and most commonly, copper. It is documented that *debens* served to compare values but were not necessarily exchanged in themselves, but items of equal value to the amount determined in debens, were exchanged. So the deben was a national unit standard of value against which all other items were valued; in other words, the value of the item was assessed in terms of debens. One deben of copper weighs between 90 and 91 grams. It was divided into ten kite (qedet or qdt).

Table 2: Approximate values of various commodities, particularly during the New Kingdom[8]

Food

1 sack of wheat (c.58 kg)	1 to 2 deben	During the latter part of the 20th dynasty, grain prices rose to between 8 and 12 deben, falling to 2 after the end of the New Kingdom. Only corn prices fluctuated thus strongly.
1 sack of barley	2 deben	
1 litre of oil	1 deben	Deir el Medina
1 jug of olive oil	1½ deben	
1 container of fresh fat	30 deben	
1 loaf of bread	0.1 deben	Deir el Medina
1 litre of beer	½ deben	
1 cake	0.2 deben	
1 litre of wine	1 deben	Deir el Medina

---

[8] http://www.touregypt.net/featurestories/prices.htm

1 thigh of a wendju cow	3½ seniu, about 30 deben	
1 bundle of vegetables	½ deben	
50 fish	2 deben	Deir el Medina
Utensils		
1 bronze kebet vessel	20 deben	
1 bronze gai vessel	16 deben	
1 pesdjet vessel	3 goldunits	
1 bronze jar	18 deben (12/3 kit of silver)	18th Dynasty
1 bronze cup	5 deben	
1 wooden sqr container	2 deben	
1 leather bucket	3 deben	
1 basket	4 deben	
Garments etc		
1 linen sheet	33 deben (31 /3 kit of silver)	18th Dynasty
10 shirts of fine linen	4 kit of silver	18th Dynasty
1 shirt	5 deben	
1 shirt	2½ deben	Deir el Medina
1 smooth DAj garment	30 deben	
1 smooth dAjw garment	11 deben	
1 smooth sDj.t garment	10 deben	
1 kalasiris	20 deben	
1 dAjw garment	20 deben	

1 pair of sandals	2 deben	
Grooming		
1 razor	2 deben	Deir el Medina
1 razor	1 deben	
1 mirror	6 deben	Deir el Medina
1 fly-swat	1 deben	Deir el Medina
1 glass-pearl necklace	5 deben	
1 amulet	1 deben	
Furniture		
1 woven mat	1 deben	
1 bed	12-20 deben	
1 chair	20 deben	
1 chair, 1 foot-stool, 1 post	13 deben	
1 table	15 deben	
1 chest	1 deben	
1 sleeping mat (?)	2 deben	
Timber		
1 DpH-wide plank of aS wood	1 kit of copper	20th Dynasty
1 Drat plank of aS wood	2 kit of silver per cubit length	20th Dynasty
Animals		
1 bird	¼ deben	Deir el Medina
1 goat	2½ deben	Deir el Medina

1 donkey	25 deben	
1 donkey	40 deben	
1 cow	up to 140 deben	
1 bull	120 deben	
1 bull	50 deben	Deir el Medina
1 ox	60 deben	Under Ramses XI

Land

lease of 1 arura	about 5 deben	11th dynasty
1 arura	0.17 deben of silver	18th dynasty
1 arura	0.5 to 0.6 deben of silver	21st dynasty
1 arura	0.1 deben of silver	21st dynasty

Funerary equipment

1 linen shroud	50 deben (5 kit of silver)	18th dynasty
1 simple wooden coffin	20-40 deben	
1 scribe's coffin	200 deben	
1 simple ushabti	0.02 deben	
1 set of simple canopic jars	5 deben	
1 'Book of the Dead'	100 deben	Deir el Medina
1 wooden statuette	10 deben	

Slaves

1 slave girl	4 deben of silver	18th dynasty
1 ordinary male slave	3 deben 1 kit of silver	21st dynasty
Metal	(Ratios are approximate)	
1 kit of gold	2 kit of silver : 1 to 2	Until the 20th Dynasty
1 kit of silver	10 deben of copper : 1 to 100	Until the 20th Dynasty
1 kit of gold	2 kit of copper : 1 to 200	Throughout the New Kingdom
1 kit of silver	6 deben of copper : 1 to 60	Late 20th Dynasty
1 kit of silver	33 deben of copper : 1 to 330	Ptolemaic Period

The passage below shows that oil and grain could serve as a kind of currency.

The Middle Kingdom priest Heqanakhte preferred to be paid in grain:

> *Concerning him who will give me payment in oil - he shall give me 1 big jar of oil for 2 sacks of Lower Egyptian barley or for 3 sacks of emmer. Behold, I prefer to be given my property as Lower Egyptian barley.*

Ancient Egyptian Economics

3rd letter of Heqanakhte
After a German translation on the *Thesaurus Linguae Aegyptiae* http://aaew.bbaw.de/tla/

Gold was not used as a standard per se in Ancient Egypt, the way it is conceived in modern times. Gold was a storehouse of physical wealth but also seen as a reflection of timeless and immortal qualities of divinity, the sun, so possessing it represented closeness to the spiritual essence of the Divine. The value ratios for the most common commodities would have been known generally, but the wide ranging value combinations brought into existence an abstract value system. Certain amounts were based on a *deben*, *seniu*[9] or, beginning with the New Kingdom, a *kit* of gold, silver and copper were used as units. Generally, no metal appears to have changed hands during the commercial exchanges until the Late Period of Ancient Egyptian history.

The use of metal rings as a standard of a given weight goes back to the Old Kingdom era of Ancient Egyptian history. Among the artifacts found in Queen Hetep-heres I's tomb was a jewel box that had the inscription:

> *Mother of the King of Upper and Lower*
> *Egypt, Hetep-heres.*
> *Box containing deben rings.*
> Reiser, George A. *The Household Furniture*
> *of Queen Hetep-heres I,*
> BMFA 27, No. 164, December 1929, pp. 83-
> 90

---

9 seniu: or shat, was used until the New Kingdom, one twelfth of a deben, about 7.6 grammes, was replaced by the kit.

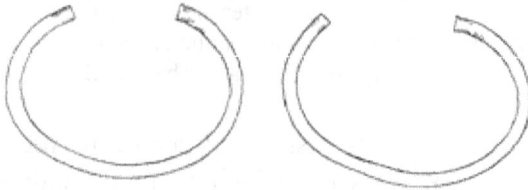

Figure 9: deben rings

Old and Middle Kingdom (about 2025-1700 BC) inscribed weights attest to units of around 12-14 grams, and 27 grams. A late Middle Kingdom account (Papyrus Boulaq 18) refers to 'small' and 'large' deben. Other sources refer to a gold deben and a copper deben. It seems likely that 1 gold deben = 12-14 grams, 1 copper deben = 27 grams[10]

The introduction of money as we know it today

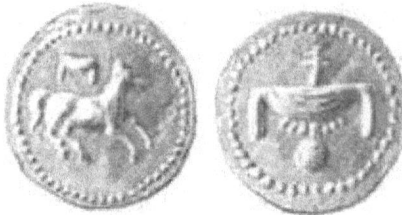

Symbols on right: "nefer nub" (good gold)
Figure 10: Ancient Egyptian coins

In the fifth century B.C.E. [early Late Period], foreign coins were being introduced to Kamit [Ancient Egypt]. In the beginning, those imported silver and gold pieces were used by the Ancient Egyptians as precious metal of standardized weight rather than true currency money. From the mid 4th century B.C.E. and onwards, as the Greek mercenaries in Egypt began demanding payment *in specie*, and as Mediterranean traders relied more

[10] http://www.digitalegypt.ucl.ac.uk/weights/weight.html

and more on coined metal as means of exchange, the Ancient Egyptian mint produced coins[11] [see above] that were similar to Athenian tetradrachms. Under the rule of the Ptolemies, coins were later struck that bared the effigies of the Hellenist [Greek] rulers.

IOU's were often written on pot shards [ostraca] or other pieces of matter that were flat enough to be written on.

> *Owed by Apahte, son of Patai: 30 pieces of*
> *silver.*
> *Written in the year 28(?), on the 30th of*
> *Mesore.*
> Demotic ostrakon, Ptolemaic Period,
> Victoria-Museum, Uppsala, inv. no. 982
> My translation from the German[12]

Aside from personal credits, the people were able to deposit grain in state warehouses and later write withdrawal orders that served as payment.[13] Instead of paying interest on the deposit, these grain banks worked by deducting 10% (*demurrage* - Compensation paid for such detention.). Some researchers theorize that due to the demurrage, the Ancient Egyptians did not need to hoard their wealth, but proceeded to keep on spending it, most often on the maintenance and improvement of the older temples and for the building of new temples. However, since the basic needs of life were provided for through collective work and distribution of goods needed for survival, there was

---

11 Coins struck in Ancient Egypt exhibit the Athenian owl, but the Greek olive branch was substituted for a papyrus plant and the inscriptions were in Aramaic or Demotic.

12 Wangstedt, Sten V. Ausgewählte demotische Ostraka aus der Sammlung des Victoria-Museums zu Uppsala und der Staatlichen Papyrussammlung zu Berlin

13 Origins of Money and of Banking by Roy Davie

no need for saving money for the purpose of developing riches or for inordinate social security needs. For example, there is evidence that excess grain from years with abundant harvests was stored for use in lean years. Also, if there was a need in one part of the country, part of the excess would be sent there. So the collective surplus was used to mitigate any shortfalls throughout the country so that no member of the society should have to suffer unnecessarily for lack of the basic necessities of life. This practice existed prior to the introduction of coin money.

Ancient Egyptian Wisdom Teachings:

> "Those who give away their treasure wisely, giveth away their plagues: they that retain their increase, heap up sorrow."

> "The earth is barren of good things where she hoards up treasure; where gold is in her bowels, there no herb grows."

> "Help your friends with the things that you have, for you have these things by the grace of God. If you fail to help your friends, one will say "you have a selfish soul". One plans for tomorrow, but you do not know what tomorrow will bring. The right soul is the soul by which one is sustained. If you do praiseworthy deeds, your friends will say "welcome" in your time of need."

During the Hellenistic (Greek) period, this banking system became a countrywide and not just a local phenomenon. Accounts were maintained at a central bank in the capital city of Alexandria and the granaries formed a financial system like the British giro[14] network.

> *Wealth accrues to him who guards it;*
> *Let your hand not scatter it to strangers,*
> *Lest it turn to loss for you.*
> *If wealth is placed where it bears interest,*
> *It comes back to you redoubled;*
> *Make a storehouse for your own wealth,*
> *Your people will find it on your way.*
> *What is given small returns augmented,*
> *[What is replaced brings abundance.]*
>
> The Instruction of Any
> M. Lichtheim *Ancient Egyptian Literature* Vol. 2, p.138f

Increasingly, now in the Greek conquest period, the banks began to deal more and more with coin money instead of perishable grain. The example below is of orders for payment crediting and debiting accounts at the royal bank of Greek-controlled Ancient Egypt:

> *[And there is a notice of payment, as*
> *payment for the honorable . . .] The form of*
> *the customary notice of payment is as*
> *follows. To be credited to the account of the*
> *sacred offices(?). Due to the king from*
> *Asklepiades son of Euphris(?), of the*
> *Zephyrian deme, as payment for the*
> *honourable office of prophet which he*
> *purchased in the temple in Menelais of the*
> *Menelaite nome, 500 drachmai(?).*
>
> P.Mich.:1:9, 257 BCE
> APIS record: michigan.apis.1864

The ancient peoples did not have identification cards and social security numbers. However, the ancient banks were concerned with positive

---

14 a British financial system in which a bank or a post office transfers money from one account to another when they receive authorization to do so

identification of people doing business at the royal bank (which actually served as a central bank). Remember that there were dire consequences for anyone defrauding the bank or committing any crime in Ancient Egypt. The bank recorded a person's ancestry, physical characteristics, age, profession and other pertinent information:

> *... through the bank of Sarapion of the Stoa of Athena. Isidoros son of Marion, to Hermas son of Heron, grandson of Hermas, from the second Goose Pen ward, aged forty years with a scar in the middle of his forehead, (acknowledges) that he (Hermas) has received from Isidoros an interest-bearing loan of a principal of one hundred twenty silver drachmas, which he will pay back in the month of Pauni of the current year forthwith.*
> *(second hand) I, Hermas, have borrowed the one hundred twenty drachmas, which I will pay back in the month of Pauni of the same ninth year, as set forth above.*
> ***P.Col.:10:259, 146 CE***
> ***APIS record: columbia.apis.p292***

In the Greek and Roman controlled era of Ancient Egypt, the money lenders were concerned about obtaining collateral when lending. The wisdom writings of Sage Ankhsheshonq (about 2nd-1st century B.C.E.) gave words of advice to all prospective lenders:

> *"Do not lend money at interest without obtaining a security."* and *"Do not be too trusting lest you become poor."*

Ankhsheshonq also had prudent advice about how borrowed money should be used by a borrower so as to make the most of the money through investment in worthwhile ventures, building its value and progressing in life, instead of squandering it in short term enjoyments:

> *Borrow money at interest and put it in farmland.*
> *Borrow money at interest and take a wife.*
> *Borrow money at interest and celebrate your birthday.*
> *Do not borrow money at interest in order to live well on it.*
>
> M. Lichtheim,
> *Ancient Egyptian Literature*, Vol.3, p.172

A person pledging their property could receive credit. Pawnbrokers did exist in Egypt, at least from the time of the Roman conquest period. Some frequent items pawned were jewelry, furniture, utensils and metal implements:

> *The bronze vessels of Claudius (?) Severus were redeemed when the report of his [property ?] was made ..... and payment was made for the interest on the bond from Epeiph of the 4th year to Tybi [of the 7th year], a period of 31 months, at the rate of 110 drachmas per month, a total 3,410 drachmas, and for the principal 1 talent 5,600 drachmas , and from Theon for the redemption of his Aphrodite 400 drachmas, amounting to 2 talents 3,410 drachmas for principal and interest. The remaining ..... four thousand six hundred drachmas, in total .... talents, 4,600 drachmas [are secured] by the remaining pledges, which are ..... a pair of armlets, a pair of cups, a pair of anklets, a necklace, a spearshaped ornament. Another cupboard was given in addition .....*
>
> **from P.Mich.inv. 1950, 3rd century CE**
> **APIS record: michigan.apis.1554**

Degeneration of the Ancient Egyptian Economy in the Late Period

The ancient system of distribution of goods throughout Ancient Egypt operated in a way so that goods were collected by royal decree and the Vizier, governors, and tax collectors and a veritable army of bureaucrats managed the process. So farm crops in the north of Egypt were collected and redistributed so that everyone would get what they needed. Crops of a different sort in the south would in turn be redistributed to the north, and so on. Therefore, this was a massive system of economy based on collective sharing of the wealth of the country without leaving some to fend for themselves or creating associations or guilds that segregate people from subsistence level goods for the sake of commercial profit. This system of economy may be thought of as a *Barter and Collective Sharing Economy*. One present day similar but small-scale system of sharing is called *Community-supported agriculture (CSA)*. Typically, CSA farms are small, independent, labor intensive, family farms.[15] In Ancient Egypt, the system was countrywide and managed by the central government, the Pharaonic system. By Roman times, however, the Pharaonic state which had controlled the general economy by collecting and redistributing had been mostly dismantled by the Roman conquerors in favor of a colonial administrative system, which had the main goal of exploiting Egypt in favor of Rome. Egypt became the "breadbasket" that allowed the Roman Empire to grow, but Egypt was depleted of its wealth.

---

15 Wikipedia, the free encyclopedia © 2001-2006

Figure 11: Barter and trading at a market in old kingdom ancient Egypt

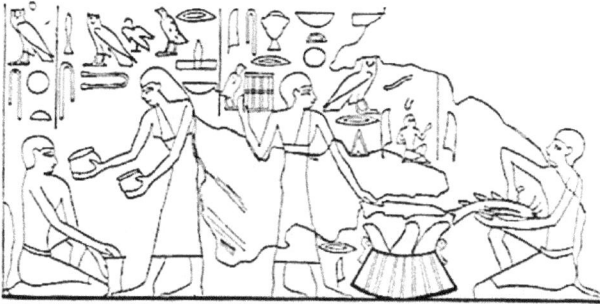

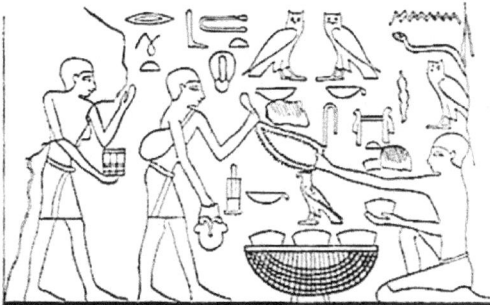

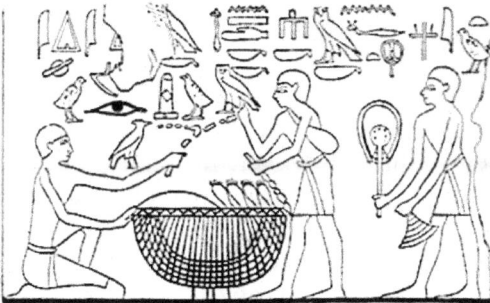

MARKETING UNDER THE OLD EMPIRE (after L. D., ii. 96).

Trade was an integral part of the Ancient Egyptian economy. The Ancient Egyptian economy was self sustaining, having all things needed to sustain the culture. However, the Ancient Egyptians traded with many surrounding countries and with other parts of Africa as well as Greece, Asia Minor and as far away as India. Trade fell under the control of private persons who often organized themselves in guilds, but the economy as a whole was supported by the Pharaoh. That change towards control of private persons may be seen as the emergence of a merchant class, an early form of what would much later be called "**bourgeoisie**", the forerunner of modern day "pseudo-capitalism"; it was a development that led to the depletion of Ancient Egyptian natural resources and to human suffering, as there began to be a large divergence between the wealthy and the general populace; so the class of the "poor" as we know it today, came into being there.

"Pseudo-capitalism" may be thought of as the application of capitalist rhetoric to what is essentially corporate socialism. It is a deception by owners of capital to cause the public at large to believe, through a propaganda network including right wing and left wing politicians, right wing television and radio commentators, that left wing or democratic critics are undemocratic and against government and capitalism,[16] and that they live in a fair system of economy where resources are distributed safely, fairly and equitably through private enterprises and where effort is rewarded fairly and equitably through hard work and or entrepreneurship. However, in reality the resources are controlled by the capitalist class and income derived from investments is disproportionately directed to the wealthy class. Capitalism theory holds that people who own capital and invest it

---

[16] One of the most prominent front persons for the powers behind the propaganda is Glen Beck, who constantly whips up fears about (unfounded) left wing conspiracies. Though he has dwindling business sponsors, he is supported by rich financiers of his programs.
http://www.democracynow.org/2011/1/14/why_is_glenn_beck_obsessively_targeting

should suffer the risk of gain and loss, but in "pseudo-capitalism" (the economic system of the U.S.A. and other countries), the losses are transferred to the masses while profits are retained by the corporations and their owners. The system of government and economics is controlled by plutocracy (rule by the wealthy class) and managed through fascism (collusion of corporations with government through plutocrat financing of government officials {congress, the president and Supreme Court} to control their actions, namely making laws in favor of the wealthy class). Capitalism theory supposes that varied parties competing would lead to some products winning; but "pseudo-capitalism" promotes control by private persons of resources needed by all and monopolies over resources, enterprises and territories, such that true competition does not occur because crony capitalism supports businesses that would otherwise lose in a real competitive environment; all of which is in contradiction with the concept of fair governance practiced in Ancient Egypt for thousands of years before. "Pseudo-capitalism" is the authorization and institutionalization of economic injustice where the economy is controlled by cabals that do not have the interests of the majority at heart. Today the cabals are controlled by the moneyed interests, those who own and or control the following industries which are the most powerful, and which contribute the most (legalized bribery) to congress, the president and the Supreme Court: the credit based banks, the prison industrial complex, the military industrial complex, the pharmaceutical industry, the health insurance industry, and the oil and energy industries. These industries may be referred to as "Cabal industries." They are the economic centers of most power and influence and are controlled by a power elite, through which they determine the wealth of a society and protect the power of their own class over the masses of all countries. Such cabals were not allowed in Ancient Egypt.

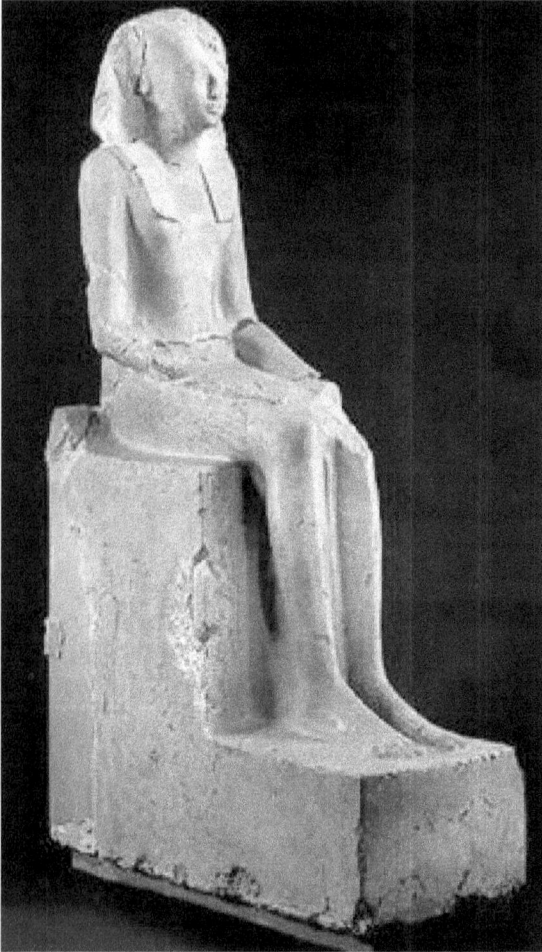

Figure 12: Pharaoh Hatshepsut. Queen Hatshepsut and other Pharaohs sent trading expeditions down the Red Sea to the Land of Punt and to other places.

On next page:
Figure 13: A Depiction from Hatshepsut's Temple Recording the Punt Expedition

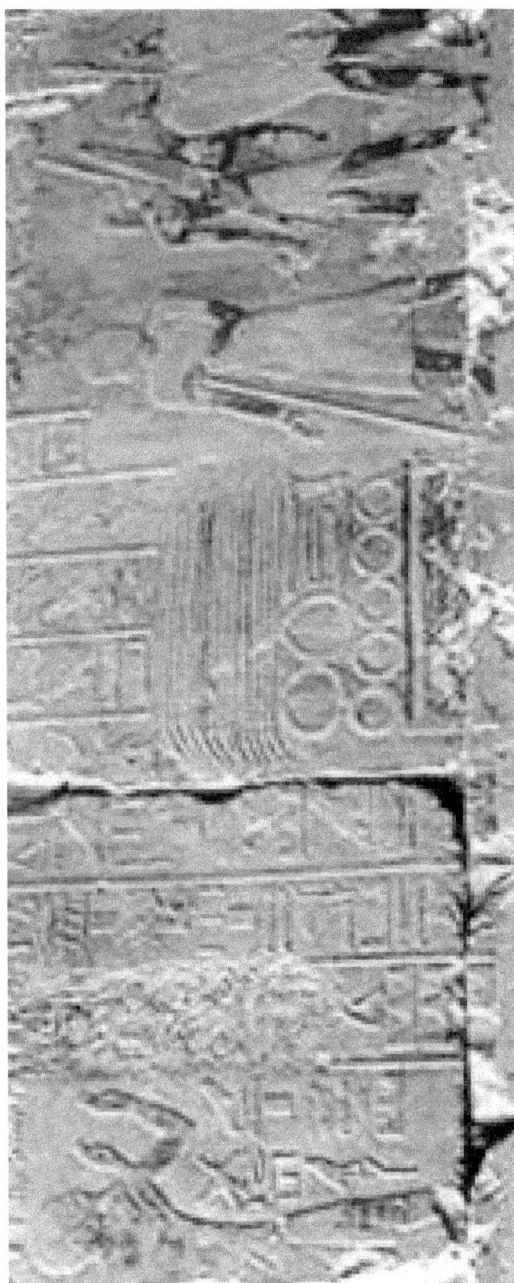

Sailors on the trading ships were paid in grain. When their ships stopped to unload, they were able to visit dockside shops to exchange their grain for clothes, fresh fruit, and vegetables. One such example is the association of the salt merchants of Tebtunis:

> *The undersigned men, salt merchants of*
> *Tebtynis, meeting together have decided by*
> *common consent to elect one of their*
> *number, a good man, Apynchis, son of*
> *Orseus, both supervisor and collector of the*
> *public taxes for the coming eighth year of*
> *Tiberius*
>
> P.Mich.:5:245, 47 CE
> APIS record: michigan.apis.2876

After the Romans conquered Egypt, a positive interest rate scheme imposed on invested capital was introduced to the economy and the wealth from the profits was taken out of the country, and so the temple sites began to decline. What occurred to Egypt at the hands of the Roman Empire recalls what recent colonial powers such as the British Empire, the other European colonial powers, and most recently, the U.S.A. have done to smaller weaker countries as well as the regions of poor people in the U.S.A. itself (internal colonialism on the poor). The guilds may be likened to today's multinational corporations in some ways. The guilds assigned territories that had special privileges. One example is the territory paid for by one Orseus. Orseus paid 66 drachmas to have a monopoly for selling gypsum in the particular region of Tebtunis.

> *(they, i.e. the merchants, have decided) that*
> *all alike shall sell salt in the aforesaid*
> *village of Tebtynis, and that Orseus alone*

has obtained by lot the sole right to sell
gypsum in the aforesaid village of Tebtynis
and in the adjacent villages,
P.Mich.:5:245, 47 CE
APIS record: michigan.apis.2876

The guilds also fixed prices. They also set and imposed fines on anyone who would undercut them:

they shall sell the good salt at the rate of two
and one-half obols, the light salt at two
obols, and the lighter salt at one and one-
half obol, by our measure or that of the
warehouse. And if anyone shall sell at a
lower price than these, let him be fined eight
drachmai in silver for the common fund and
the same for the public treasury;
P.Mich.:5:245, 47 CE
APIS record: michigan.apis.2876

CONCLUSION

This very brief overview displays the Ancient Egyptian system of economy and how the Greek and Roman conquerors changed it into an early form of capitalist [imperialist] economy that eventually failed with the downfall of the Greco-Roman cultures. It is interesting to note that the Ancient Egyptian culture lasted for thousands of years [Ancient Egyptian economic system: 5,000-10,000 years] while the Greco-Roman cultures only existed for a few hundred years.

Ancient Egyptian economics was based on providing for human needs of the whole population within a context of a trust between the *heka* (Pharaoh) and the *hekat* (populace). While there were wealthy people in Ancient Egypt, there were no super rich or fabulously wealthy people and that allowed more wealth to be spread among the

47

population more evenly. In Ancient Egypt the Pharaoh was responsible for the people's well being and that meant that he or she could not favor the wealthy over the less wealthy nor could they allow people to become so poor as to live in hunger or languish in destitution. Enshrined in one of the main documents of Ancient Egyptian duty is the injunction to provide food, shelter and opportunity for all. So, the favoritism and disparity between the wealthy and the poor that has developed in so called capitalist or market economies would be rejected as unjust and inhumane. This means that the concepts of capitalism and consumerism are to be rejected in favor of economic systems that provide for the common good, not just for the citizens of one's own country, but the citizens of all countries. Ancient Egyptian society was not based on imperialism, so there was no need to raise vast armies for conquest and occupation of other lands. Polluters were punished by law, so the environment was protected for future generations. Imagine if the Ancient Egyptians had despoiled the environment on the scale that modern culture has done, what would we have now? Answer: an unsustainable ecology.[17]

The Ancient Egyptian system of economics was not based on perpetual expansion of the "GROSS DOMESTIC PRODUCT" and fiat currency but rather on sustainability. This means that there would be no boom or bust periods or inflation and loss of value, but rather a balanced and steady predictable economy where all members of the society have a place and the value of wealth is maintained from generation to generation for the benefit of all and not just the wealthy few.

---

[17] see the books *Egyptian Book of the Dead* and *Introduction to Maat Philosophy* by Muata Ashby

PART 2: THE PHILOSOPHY OF KEMETIC ECONOMICS

A Conversation with Sebai MAA on the Principles and Philosophy of Kemetic Economics

The following is a transcript of an interview in which Dr. Muata Ashby (Sebai MAA) expressed the fundamental philosophical underpinnings of Ancient Egyptian Economic theory and practice. The bold sections of text were questions posed to Dr. Ashby.

What are the principles of Kemetic Economics? And how can they be implemented today to help us deal with our own finances and the turbulent economies of the world today?

These teachings span different periods of Ancient Egyptian history. The earliest ones were from the Old Kingdom era which is after the Pyramid Texts era and these go all the way down through into the Late Period, which is about 4,000 years later.

There are two ways that these principles that I'm going to talk about now are to be implemented; one way is as an individual and the other, as a group. For those who may be reading this or who are in a different country, be it the Caribbean or Europe or Africa or wherever, or those who are here in this country acting as individuals, these principles ought to be applied to their best possible capacity. If there are others in your same area where you can have a group, the principles can be applied even more effectively because you can do more things effectively when people are cooperating.

First of all, it's important to understand that Ancient Egyptian society was guided by the principles of ⬧𒑱 Ma'at (Maat) philosophy. Ma'at is founded on the principle of cosmic order, of balance, of truth. In reference to this topic that we're talking about, Ma'atian philosophy states, in the PertmHeru text Chapter 125, that the poor of a society or really everyone in a society is to be taken care of and in three fundamental ways, at least, at the minimum.

> "Be generous as long as you live. What leaves the storehouse does not return. It is the food in the storehouse that one must share, that is coveted. One whose belly is empty becomes an opponent. Therefore, do not have an accuser or an opponent as a neighbor. Your kindness to your neighbors will be a memorial to you for years."
> -Ancient Egyptian Proverb

The text further states that the hungry need to be fed, the clothless need to be clothed and those who are boatless need to be given a boat, which means that if you do not have the means to feed yourself, you are to be fed. You're supposed to have the basic needs of life taken care of if you live in a righteous and balanced society. And this is done for practical purposes as well as for moral/ethical/spiritual considerations.

It is stated, in the Ancient Egyptian Proverbs, that if you have a hungry person, that person is going to be angry, that person is going to be agitated and violent. You're going to have disruption in the order of society so you need to make sure everyone who's hungry is fed, everyone who's clothless is clothed, and give a boat to the boatless (opportunity), meaning that if a person cannot acquire the basic items for sustenance of life, food, clothing, shelter and opportunity, these things should be provided by the community. Only then you can have peace and harmony in the society, because people's basic needs are going to be taken care of, and the pressure and anxiety over the lack of basic sustenance will not cause people to turn to base feelings, desires or become low of character, sufficiently to turn to crime or other unethical acts that cause harm to society.

Then they can work on higher order things, like educating themselves, like working on a skill, exploring the meaning of life and so on and so forth. So those are the foundations of Ma'at philosophy for social order. There are two wings of Ma'at philosophy, shall we say.

One is dedicated to social order as the foundation to a righteous society and the other wing is dedicated towards spiritual enlightenment and you have to have one before you can have the other. Social order and peace are needed in order to have a righteous environment conducive to spiritual advancement. Social order is based in equity and fairness in the distribution of resources. So this means that capitalism and consumerism, pollution and poverty cannot be allowed in a righteous society that wants to encourage the positive human capacities. It's interesting that, in reference to the concept of poverty, as of this writing, there are 40 million people in the United States who are on food stamps, who would otherwise be hungry. That is about 20 percent of the population.

And that's a disgrace for a country that is supposed to be the most powerful or richest in the world. It's nonsense. It's interesting that Mother Teresa visited the USA once and she experienced the extremes of wealth between rich and poor and she said that she had not witnessed the kind of poverty that she had seen here compared to in India where people are extremely poor in India, even living on the street; so the kind of poverty that people have in the USA is even worse, especially considering the greater material abundance. This points to disgraceful callousness, insensitivity and uncaring nature of the wealthy as well as the suffering, resentment and the feelings of loss, by the poor, of not being able to share in the wealth of the rest of the country. This is further shameful due to being a country with a majority that supposedly espouses the principles of Christianity: "Love thy neighbor as thyself".

"Eat not bread if another is suffering want, and thou dost not stretch out the hand to him with bread....One is rich and another is poor. He that was rich in past years is this year a groom. Be not greedy about filling the belly. The course of the water of last year, it is this year in another place. "
      -Sage Ani (Ancient Egyptian Wisdom Texts)

Along with that, you have the idea of philanthropy where the rich are supposed to give away some of their wealth. This partial giving may allow the wealthy to sleep at night, to ease their conscience, thinking they have done some good towards alleviating suffering. But what about the systematic injustice of an economic system that benefits the wealthy to begin with? A system that causes and perpetuates the suffering in the first place? Well, what if we had an ethically ordered society, then there would be no need for philanthropy because that would be taken care of by everyone as a group, a community, everyone taking care of everyone else by sharing the burden of life and also providing an opportunity for everyone via the common resources that individuals would to be able to access in order to provide for themselves. There would be no need to see people develop hardheartedness, despair, ignorance, self-deprecation and engage in self-destructive behaviors through feelings of inadequacy and inferiority; all of which leads to hatred, violence, insanity, depression and general unhappiness.

In countries like the USA, the societal philosophy dictates a kind of society where one is made to struggle, supposedly so that one will have an incentive to strive, to produce, etc. It is a clever devise used as an excuse to withhold resources from people so that others may hoard and benefit from them. While people can be motivated to struggle by making them suffer, I think that human beings don't need that kind of extra stress in order to strive. A negative aspect of that kind of striving is a movement towards resentment against society that leads to anger, hatred, crime and greed that eat away at the fabric of society, and thus diminish the capacity for advancement of a society since the people that would otherwise be working for the advancement of society would be presently working to chip away at its constructions through lack of cooperation with others in society, disparagement of the social order and even crime against society and its members. I mean that people naturally want to strive, especially when they see opportunity to progress, make things better for themselves and people prefer ethical means of doing better if that is available. I think each of us prove that, and other societies have also proven that. For example, Ancient Egyptian culture produced great works in art, architecture, philosophy, religion, law, government, and science without those kinds of negative incentives. How did they achieve that success? They achieved it by creating a balanced and just society that allows its members to naturally seek for what is beneficial and altruistic while not having to worry about the basic necessities of life; and of course, the entire society had the opportunity to strive for the greatest human achievement possible, *nehast* spiritual enlightenment, through the extensive temple system, as opposed to the perishable and ultimately unsatisfying goal of physical riches. The restriction of resources in an unrighteous society is not just for the purpose of creating an incentive, but rather an excuse for the hoarding of wealth by the rich segment of society, which allows them to exercise

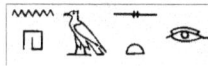

55

control over the economy, directing it to their own benefit, but also maintaining control over the members of the society, to keep them in line through dependence upon them and their rationing of the resources, all with an illusory incentive of somehow striking it rich one day, or at least becoming financially capable of having some desires fulfilled, such as getting an expensive car, going to the superbowl or world cup, meeting a Hollywood star, traveling to Europe, etc.

The following Ancient Egyptian tomb inscriptions were carved into the walls of those people who professed to have lived a righteous and orderly life. Central to this order and virtue are the acts of righteousness, and the highest form of right action is selfless service to humanity, that is, all of the things a person can do to uphold truth, order and righteousness during their lives. These inscriptions demonstrate devotion for social justice as a requisite for attaining spiritual emancipation.

❶

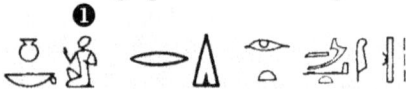

Nuk rdy maat
Give righteousness order and truth to humanity

❷

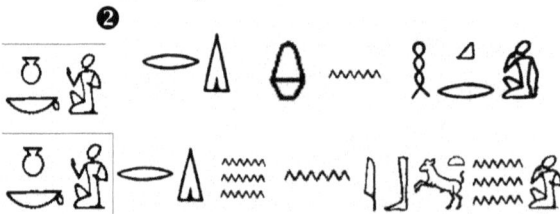

Nuk rdy ta n heqer - Nuk rdy mu n abt

56

Give food to the hungry - Give water to the thirsty

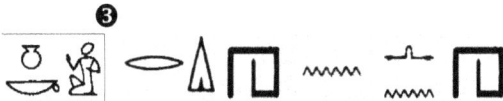

❸

Nuk rdy het n an het
Give shelter to the homeless

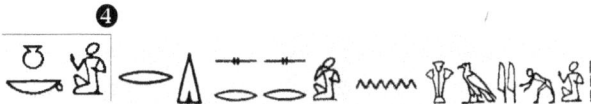

❹

Nuk rdy serser n haiu
Give comfort to the weepers (suffering-disheartened)

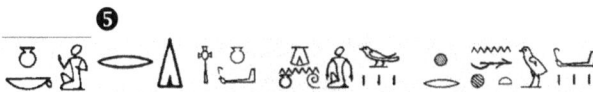

❺

Nuk rdy netu genu kher nekhtu
Give protection to the weak from the strong

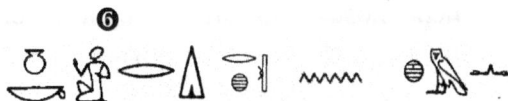

❻

Nuk rdy rech n kheman
Give wisdom (counsel) to the ignorant

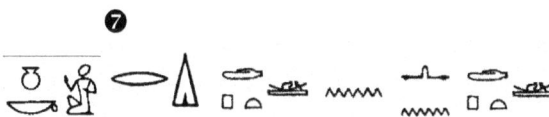

❼

Nuk rdy dept n an dept

Give opportunity to the discouraged

Items 2, 3, and 7 are specifically admonished in the PertmHeru text (Book of Enlightenment).[18] These inscriptions demonstrate the ideal observed by members of the Ancient Egyptian society. With such impetus, the societal philosophy dictated service to humanity and true caring for the well-being of the members of the society over concerns such as profit, or negative motivations.

How is the prison industrial complex, as a business or as a corporation, morally unjust and how does it contribute to the decay of the society?

Muata Ashby: Well, this matter is central to the issue of righteous and effective economics because when people are forced to live in a state of poverty or near poverty, many people become disappointed, angry and unethical. Many also turn to stealing and even violence. The provocation of stress and strife overwhelms their sense of ethical conscience. Then those who are in control or beholden to those who are (the wealthy and powerful) have a ready solution, police and military to keep people in line, and laws that maintain their subservience and keep their civil rights impaired; Legislators maintain control also through unfair tax policies that keep the masses from gaining wealth, unfair access to education that keep the masses from

---

[18] Commonly referred to as: Ancient Egyptian Book of the Dead

gaining wisdom about life and how to gain independence from financial controllers and unfair access to social upward mobility, since those positions are occupied and controlled by the moneyed interests. This problem is exacerbated by processing through the legal system, which attaches criminal records that prevent a person from getting good jobs or fully participating in the political field either as voters or candidates, thereby insuring that the class which has most of the social support (the wealthy) will have the greater opportunities and the capacity to maintain the status quo. Keep in mind that since the inauguration of Ronald Reagan as president of the USA there has been a concerted effort to keep limited access to education, keep wages down, destroy labor unions and shift the burden of taxes away from the rich and the corporations to the middle class and the poor. These policies have been referred to as *Reaganomics.* However, prior to Reagan's inauguration, the process of undercutting the masses had begun. From 1820-1970 worker wages had risen along with the rise in income of the rich. This pattern fueled the ideal of the "American Dream" and faith in the USA economic model (except for periods like the Great Depression). Most people thought that they would do better than the generation before them. However, in the 1970s, inflation due to excessive borrowing by the government for unethical expenses such as the Viet Nam War caused prices to rise. At the same time corporations stopped raising wages, seeing that people would work more since they were convinced that "times were hard".

This period was at the time of the massive introduction of computers and robots to do the work that people had done previously. Worker output (production per worked hours) increased dramatically; companies made more profit than at any other time in US history. Yet workers were not compensated more for being more productive. Also, immigration caused a glut of workers. So owners of corporations saw they could take their pick of workers (low demand for labor), in other words, take advantage of them; then came the time of outsourcing of jobs, moving factories overseas to capture low wage workers in developing countries. This left workers in the USA with lower wages and needing to send other members of the family to go to work to bring in the same income and maintain the same wasteful, gluttonous American lifestyle, a process which is still ongoing today. Yet that still was not enough, so people began to live on credit cards and home equity loans from the artificially inflated economy (inflated with the same money that corporation owners saved from not paying workers). They invested those funds and artificially caused bubbles in the economy. So the apparent wealth that people thought they had in their homes (home equity loans) was illusory; yet the owners of the mortgages want it to still be paid back. Again, this is the wealth gained by now not paying workers rising wages, unlike previous generations, and loaned back to them and expected to be paid back with interest! (Wealth that should have belonged to the workers through normally rising wages was given as a loan) some have characterized this phase of capitalism in history as "capitalism gone wild," wildly outrageous and rampantly in favor of the rich without any concern for the rest of the population or the economy as a whole. Prior to Reaganomics, the average debt was 30% of annual income; in 2007 it was 130%. So the middle and lower classes of the US population is so in debt and the US government is so in debt that it has led to an unprecedented situation where, having lost the manufacturing base (was outsourced to other countries) there are no good prospects for recovery of the economy based on fundamentals of the economy.[19]

Such a condition would not have been allowed by the Ancient Egyptians, as there was no allowance of private ownership of capital in forms that would hurt the country; this is against Maat regulations. This form of government/socio-economic order of the USA has been referred to as "neo-feudalism" (new feudal system), a process in which people are turned into serfs; in effect. In medieval Europe, a serf was a person bound to the land owned by a lord and passed on to a new lord who purchased that land, and bound to the next lord in perpetual servitude. Today the serfdom (slavery) is one of economic destitution and the lords are the wealthy plutocrats. As a result the middle class has been severely reduced and the poor have increased, but also the percentage of the population that is incarcerated has increased to the point where the USA is the country with the largest population of

---

19 *Capitalism Hits the Fan: The Global Economic Meltdown and What to Do About It* Richard Wolff

incarcerated people in the world. Essentially, a prison industrial complex is a corporate sector of the economy, and is sanctioned by government leaders who receive legalized bribes from the corporations (campaign donations) that profit from having people in jail or being detained, (illegal immigrants, detaining convicts or arrested persons). Whenever you have a corporate or profit motive interest, be it in your health care, in your penal system, or in anything, generally, you're going to have corruption because the morals of the people are going to deteriorate such that they are going to unrighteously detain others or pay off government officials to make laws that allow them to detain others (regardless of the morality of those laws) so they can be paid for that detention. Ancient Egyptian society operated with the opposite understanding, that fairness and freedom caused people to feel good about their lives and were more productive. The Wisdom Text of MeriKaRa speaks directly to this issue:

> (23) When free men are given land,
> They work for you like a single team;
> No rebel will arise among them,

For instance, corporations have been caught red-handed plotting to bribe lawmakers, Congress people to change laws so that there would be a lower minimum amount of drugs that a person has to be caught with such that there can be more people being caught and detained so they can make more of a profit. It will be better for their (the corporation's) bottom line, not thinking about the lives of those people or how that'll affect the society as a whole. It's a very short-sighted egoistic society that does not see the whole. That is the big difference with an evolved and righteous society, it sees the human society as a whole, as a body, with equally valuable members and not as individuals who are to be exploited.

And that's on one side, the corporate side. On the empire side, that is, the American Empire, it is important for the empire to be able to incarcerate enough people to have a deterrent against dissent but also, and perhaps more importantly, crime (which would disrupt corporate activities-interrupt business hours). It is also important to have the capacity of processing (detaining and marking) certain members of the population so that their activities can be controlled, their political aspirations that would challenge the corporate state can be thwarted, their upper mobility can be limited and so on. The police and the army therefore become agents for the oligarchy, for the corporatists, the rich people to keep the society in check, to keep the masses in check and keep other countries in check. It becomes more important to have an industrial level penal system for a large unrighteous country, in a society that forces people to live in ways that we've just discussed that are unrighteous and that do not take care of their basic needs because that'll force them into a life of crime. It'll force them through stress to seek other forms of relief like drugs, so the society as a whole is complicit but the most complicit are the people who control and direct society. Therefore, poverty, suffering and incarceration, to the levels that we have seen in the USA, are not an accident; it is actually the level accepted as necessary in order to achieve the levels of wealth for the economic elites (power elites, moneyed interests, the rich, etc.). In other words, the levels of poverty and incarceration are a direct effect of the levels of desired economic disparity that will allow a minority to have most of the wealth and power of society. Such a system was unheard of in Ancient Egypt. There was crime and punishment but punishment was administered to the extent needed for rehabilitation; not just as a punitive measure. Also there was extensive effort towards crime prevention by promoting justice and equity in the society.

"Punish firmly and chastise soundly, then repression of crime becomes an example. But punishment except for crime will turn the complainer into an enemy."

-Ancient Egyptian Proverb

One more thing, it is important to understand that when we speak of power elites, moneyed interests, the rich, etc. we are referring to a segment of the population that live in their own special neighborhoods. I am not speaking of gated communities; those are for the upper middle class. I am speaking of the very rich. They have their own neighborhoods segregated from the rest of the population. They have their own schools, airports, supermarkets and malls, television and radio stations and have no contact with the rest of the country except when servants and maintenance personnel are allowed to come into their areas. These are the type of people that are so rich that their television stations have programs designed for them, for example, to let them know how to tell whether a diamond necklace is worth 10 million or 50 million, so they won't make a silly mistake on their next birthday gift to themselves. That kind of physical separation allows them to live in their own world, a bubble where they do not feel or see the way the masses live and that makes it easier for them to act in selfish and abusive ways without seeing the faces of their victims. They have their representatives, the lawyers, congress and senators for that lowly dirty work.

So, now given the Ma'atian principles, the foundation for a social order that you mentioned - the hungry need to be fed, the clothless need to be clothed, transportation, a boat given to the boatless - how do we take that Ma'atian foundation of the past? How do we apply these principles to today, based upon the circumstances that we have at present?

Muata Ashby: Well, firstly, those who find themselves as individuals, living in their own city, in their own country and even if there are no other followers of similar mind or of similar tradition that they can join with or they can cooperate with, they can try to apply some of these principles to their

65

capacity, as individuals. Those who are in closer proximity with others, they would be able to have more of a cooperative effort to pool their resources, pool their efforts to be able to take actions that will protect them if some negative eventuality would occur.

When two or more people make an investment, it's more powerful than if one person makes an investment alone because two people have double resources to invest, and so the outcome can be accelerated, the outcome can be heightened. So that's something that I think everyone should consider especially as we move forward; and there seems to be some time to prepare. Since I've been lecturing on this theme, (since 2006 with the publication of the book *Collapse of* Civilization) several unprecedented events have occurred but none point to economic recovery before major downward movement in the economy. The thing that we do not have exact is the timing, the timing of when these downfalls will occur. But we have knowledge and intellectual understanding of what is going to happen and how it can happen and how it's likely to happen based on the current actions of people today and on similar occurrences of the past. The modern world certainly has not followed a sound model of economics, such as was employed in Ancient Egypt. We do not know of any periods in Ancient Egyptian history that can be characterized as economic depressions, market crashes, massive, chronic unemployment or banking schemes, bailouts or inflation because there were no greedy bankers and there was no faux economy based on fiat currency and fractional banking; and of course there was no capitalism or fascism[20].

I'd like to speak of teachings related to business and commerce that I thought would bring forth the most important principles of Kemetic economics. I also think these will be very useful teachings that people can use right now. These are teachings from Sage Amenemope and from other sages.

Do not assess a man who has nothing and thus falsify your pen. If you find the large debt against a poor man, make it into three parts - forgive two and let one stand. You will find it a path of life. Haste not to be rich but be not slothful in thine own interest. One does not run to reach success; one does not move to spoil it. Don't make yourself a ferry on the river and then strain to seek its fare. Take the fare from him who is wealthy and let pass him who is poor.

I think this particular teaching embodies the highest ideals of Kemetic economics. Firstly, what about taking things from people who don't have means to protect themselves or their property? How many times have we seen people in this culture, with a stroke of a pen, taking away a person's property or their house and say, "oh, it was just business. I didn't mean it personally, it's just

---

[20] corporations and government officials colluding to make laws favorable to businesses at the expense of the general population.

business. And business is business". That higher regard of business as opposed to human beings is supposed to be a virtue but it is actually a callous business ideal espoused by those who are sociopaths or those who follow them, people who have deluded consciences; these are people that have a conscience that is tainted, contaminated by the corporate culture, people who are generally "good" but who may allow certain unrighteous behavior of themselves or others for personal gain; they tell themselves that the corporate culture is ethical even though every day we see that it is not. It is unfair. The Wisdom Text of MeriKaRa speaks directly to this issue:

> (12) You will endure on earth when you do justice;
> Calm those who weep, don't oppress the widow who is grieving,
> Don't drive out a man from the property of his father...

The people who follow the corporate culture are themselves complicit in the unrighteousness of it. Maat philosophy precludes the possibility of the emergence of a corporate culture in a Maatian society because the foundation of Maat is based on not hurting others, not hoarding wealth and not favoring certain members of society over others in business opportunities or in relation to social justice. This Maatian ideal is diametrically opposed to the corporate culture, which seeks to gain at the expense of others and the environment. Another example is turning off people's heat in the winter time, due to non-payment.

Partly, this is, I think, a product of a culture of greed and extreme libertarian values; the idea that people should fend for themselves and if they make it, fine; if they don't fine, that's extremely callous and unfeeling in such a way that it becomes a detriment to that same person's (libertarian) capacity to attain balance and order and peace in their own life. That ideal is also often coupled with capitalism to form a potent poli-economics (political/economic) philosophy that promotes apparent individualism but allows capitalist cabals to form that abuse the masses under the rubric of promoting "capitalism" (which is all good and has no negative effects) and or "individual rights". Libertarianism and capitalism are ideologies that cannot and do not work for all members of a population. Therefore they are illegitimate but most often espoused by people of means. Thus they are fundamentally unfair systems of poli-economics. So, neither greed nor libertarianism or capitalism are viable forms of socioeconomic systems for a viable, balanced and well adjusted society.

The development of the "Tea Party", a far right winged segment of the population, and other groups who are screaming the loudest about too much government spending and or about there being too many laws, are people who in their own lives are unable to find peace, they are unable to find balance and order; they are also fearful of losing their income and wealth but also, they care more about themselves than other members of the society. They also lack understanding or compassion for others. Usually you'll find that when people are screaming and accusing others, that they are the ones practicing or supporting those things that they're complaining about, that there are supposedly fearful about. So it is not surprising that we find that the so called "Tea Party" is very small but heavily funded by corporations and very rich donors who want to hide behind vocal ignorant members of the middle or lower classes who have been convinced, often through incitement of fear, to be opponents of government since that strengthens their (corporations and very rich donors) capacity to get laws that are lenient as far as regulations and prosecution for lawbreaking. Those laws are good for the corporations but unfavorable to the individuals, the same vocal ignorant members of the middle or lower classes, yet the ignorant follow out of fear, greed and ignorance.

You know, we can find a lot of politicians who complain against gays or sex scandals and then they are the ones who are found doing most of that, of being gays and being involved in sex scandals, malfeasance, etc., especially the Republicans. They accuse others of being homosexual or of stealing, later it comes out that they're the ones who turn out to have been stealing all along or who are gay, etc. They also use the subject they are ranting about to rally the segments of the population that are most ignorant, and vulnerable to fears and insecurities; this is sometimes referred to as demagoguery. A preferred tactic is to use vitriolic language to demonize and delegitimize the other groups who

70

have differences of opinion so as to have the prevailing ideology and therefore also the most accepted ideology, no matter how failed the policies based on those ideologies may be, since the followers do not look at that critically but rather with blind acceptance, in a similar way that they follow religion, with blind faith.

Going back to our proverb, so how do you handle a loan if someone cannot pay you? It says: if you divide the loan into three parts, you forgive two and keep the one. And this is what should be done with the present day real estate debacle. Those who cannot pay should have their mortgage reduced by two-thirds at least, if for no other reason, because the way that the real estate values were inflated artificially (economic bubble) by the banks and the US Federal Reserve. Due to the fraud perpetrated by banks, all loans made during that period should be adjusted likewise. This gives you an understanding of how to handle this problem. Yet, it is interesting to note the extent of the greed of heads of corporations and government leaders, who allowed the banks to operate with impunity, that is at such a level that the perpetrators of the colossal scam would be willing to continue defrauding the economy even now and let the country and the economy go down while allowing even more foreclosures, even from where we are today, rather than force the banks to take the losses and fix the laws so that it could not happen again. The debacle was their fault in the first place because not only did the bankers engage in unethical behavior creating derivative financial products they knew were unsound but also the original mortgage loans that the derivatives were based on were created fraudulently to begin with. An FBI study found that as many as 80% of the subprime mortgage loans that were given were based on fraud by the lenders, not the borrowers; fraud such as bank officers changing information to make people qualify. Yet, even though the bankers were responsible for massive losses they got lawmakers to bail them out. This is a hallmark of "pseudo-capitalism": corporate welfare. No one went to jail over the deliberate swindling of the economy. This is another hallmark of "pseudo-capitalism": impunity for high level government and corporate officials as they break laws, but stiff penalties and jail time for the masses.

It seems there was a sense of balance in Kemetic economics. What is the nature of that balance?

Muata Ashby: That's the key. It's a concept of Ma'atian balance and order where you're not going to allow yourself to be controlled by unrighteous behaviors elicited by others or your own unrighteous desires that want to lead you astray. The most important thing for a follower of Kemetic economics to work on is finding the balance between providing for the necessities of the physical life and providing for the necessities of the spiritual life. You see, if you run after things, you are controlled by those things as well as the demands that those things impose on you. If you're going after riches, you're running after fame or whatever it might be, you're controlled by those things. You are forced to do the things that you perceive are in line with attaining those things and thereby your destiny is mapped out not by your choice but by the dictates of the objects you are after. In order to lead a balanced life, you do not run after riches or objects, but you do not run away from them either. You do your duties, act responsibly and cooperatively with others, and then you let life take its course; doing this will provide for the necessities of life and will provide opportunities to make the best of life, that is, the opportunity to be truly fulfilled in life. True fulfillment does not and cannot come from attaining objects or wealth but a certain amount of wealth is necessary so that a person can have a peaceful and sane capacity to discover the purpose of their life and thus, the means to find what one needs in order to discover abiding happiness and contentment.

> *"An immoderate desire of riches is a poison lodged in the mind. It contaminates and destroys everything that was good in it. It is no sooner rooted there, than all virtue, all honesty, all natural affection, fly before the face of it."*
> -Ancient Egyptian Proverb

So anytime you're going after something, that something is controlling you, would you expand upon that?

Muata Ashby: Well, it's very simple. When you have desires, desires are based on your *ariu,* or the sum total of your feelings, your thoughts, and your experiences of the past that forms the basis for the way that you think and act today. So if you have grown up, say, in a family of musicians, it's likely that you will be growing up to like music and to desire to be a musician especially since the musician experience would be central in your upbringing and would influence your thoughts and feelings from early on. If you have those feelings from an internal force, say, because you liked music in a previous life, then the inner and outer forces strongly compel you to move in that direction and likely have great success as well. In any case, whether your desire arises out of a previous lifetime or the present one, regardless, you will be impelled towards that desire and if the basis is strong enough you will be compelled to do what is required to achieve the desire. That impel-ation and compellation is the aspect that controls a person. The intensity of the desire determines the level of impel-ation and compellation and whether or not the person can control themselves or not. That basis in a person's unconscious that determines the desires, thought and feelings of a person is what is called *ariu.*

So, if your *ariu* is to search for wealth or search for riches or fame or whatever it might be, you will pursue that; you will go after that. So this proverbial teaching is saying that one should, rather find the balance, not run towards or away from objects and let them come of their own accord, based on necessity or for sound investment. In that way, one can have peace as one pursues one's goals in life.

Finally, I would say that people should not feel disheartened about the current condition; you know, things go up and they go down. We are currently in a depressive phase of macro economics, the economics of countries. However, one need not have depression in micro economics, in one's own individual life, if there is preparation and balance in life. The important thing is to take action, to prepare, and that action will allow one to survive and to move forward. Remember that there will be another side to this, you know, once the economy bottoms out, even if there is a huge calamity, like the devastation of a war or things like that, there will be recovery. Sometimes wars also tend to be part of the mix when societies falter because that's how people can be deceived or they can be distracted away from thinking about deceptive or corrupt leaders and or failed economic systems. You can see that we already have wars that have been forgotten in this debate of the economy but people should realize that there can be worse calamities. However, other societies, other peoples have gone through worse and through darker times from the standpoint of their physical well-being and their safety. Though, not all will make it through, for want of preparation, so all should do what is in their power to protect themselves from those possible calamities.

I'm especially thinking about war torn situations and war zones and think of those people that experienced that, and we don't have that here yet so the time should be used to prepare one's finances, prepare one's self psychologically and in understanding the depth of the situation in order to make sense of it. Because when one makes sense of things, then one can have relief of stress and take responsibility and then one can take action; through that, sound thinking, courage and righteous action can come in.

But when people are ignorant, when they don't know what's happening and what may happen or what may not happen and may feel powerless, they start going either to, pledge allegiance to any demagogic leader that plays on their weak minds, showing them what other group is their enemy, or put their head in a hole or they bind together with others out of fear so that they can blame others or lash out or act self-destructively. But it's more important to find answers and to find understanding because that leads to solutions, if not for the whole society at least for individuals who will hopefully then be in a position to affect society in a larger way, in a grander and positive way when society is able to listen and take their lead.

Dr. Ashby, you have assigned a term "pseudo-capitalism", to the current system of economics used by the USA. Before going forward with Ancient Egyptian Economics could you discuss your analysis of USA economics and the American Empire so we can have a basis of comparison for what we have today versus what existed in the past and thereby we can better understand how we should move forward, and what system of economics we need and should work to establish?

Muata Ashby: it is useful to compare and contrast the economic system of Ancient Egypt with that of western countries today in order to gain a deeper understanding about what existed in ancient times and the nature of beneficial political and economic systems versus corrupt political and economic systems. Now, in reference to the issue of "pseudo-capitalism" and it's inability to provide a viable economy, many times commentators refer to our current economic system as being "broken" since it is seen as a method by which the United States of America was able to amass fantastic wealth; but in recent years its faults, like destruction of the environment and hostility towards other countries, have come into focus. Furthermore, it seems that eventually it will collapse. Additionally, there is the question, wealth for whom? It is important to understand that the economic system that may be referred to as "pseudo-capitalism" that is used in the U.S.A. is completely opposed to that which was developed in Ancient Egypt. It was created to benefit certain members of the society, the aristocracy, and today we refer to this system as plutocracy, rule by and for the rich; but they do this through corporate power and bribery of government officials. So actually, its current manifestation may more accurately be described as *"fascism"*, the administration where government and corporate power collude for the benefit of the rich at the expense of the middle class and poor masses. From its inception it was never broken since it was designed to do exactly what it has allowed the power elite of the society to accomplish, amass fantastic fortunes at the expense of the masses. In that sense it really cannot be fixed. It really has to be revamped or it has to be redone, but even that would be only a start; for even the most ethical system of government and economics can be corrupted if the people that run it and participate in it are unethical and corrupt.

For instance, you can write over a new constitution to say that the banks cant do what they're doing and the president cant go around attacking everyone or making war wherever he wants, etc., but if you're going to have a culture that is based on a philosophy of greed then all of your efforts and all your laws are going to fail because eventually people are going to corrupt them or they're going to ignore them, for personal or party gain, just as it's happening now. This is a problem of societal ethics, in other words, corrupted social ethics wherein the members of the society are generally, distorted, twisted by egoistic desires and comprehensive ignorance about the nature and meaning of life as well as ignorance about the possibility of spiritual enlightenment, an achievement that if attained, towers over all other achievements and does indeed render potentially egoistic and unrighteous, selfish characters into noble leaders and paragons of virtue; an occurrence that would put worldly affairs into a proper perspective, for service to humanity, to alleviate all suffering and for the extension of compassion and peace as opposed to the accumulation of power and wealth or the support of evanescent political ideologies or ignorant faith-based fundamentalist religiosity. There was much talk about the president George W. Bush policy of attacking Afghanistan to impose democracy on its people and the critics were saying that democracy can't be imposed; it must grow out of the people's desire to have it. It would seem that after 10 years of war and occupation the critic's point of view would be the correct one. In the same way, the people of the USA cannot easily accept fair and just government and economics because they are used to and desirous of the culture of greed that they themselves want to partake in, be it at the level of having a nice car and house and plasma TVs, etc. or be it at the level of billionaires even if it means that the USA population must hoard the wealth of the world and consume more than any other people on earth, depriving them of wealth and the conveniences of modern technology. The leaders and the people are corrupt and it would take much time and effort to change the culture of greed. Thus, the present outcome is the fruition of what was set in motion by the European settlers whose descendants setup this government and economic system. It was inevitable that it would develop into what it is, for what is fostered and supported is what develops; whatever a society's philosophy upholds, that is what will be cultivated and the succeeding generations will follow and apply it's tenets even more strongly and blindly due to being inculcated with it from an early age. So, societies, like individuals, should be careful in supporting policies or ideas that may take on a life of their own and have unintended and dire consequences later on. In this case, the societal philosophy was and is one of greed, crime, despotism, imperialism, and consumerism; this is what the US Constitution promotes and allows so this is what people will do until it can no longer be done, for whatever reason.

Dr. Ashby, could you also explain the term "societal philosophy" and how it relates?

In one of my books, *Comparative Mythology*, I talked about a concept called *"societal philosophy."* Societal philosophy is the fundamental idea or concept of purpose that a society is based upon. And the United States, for all its ideals of being a country based on Christian principles and secular ethics and so on, is really is based on greed. It's based on the ideal of being able to get rich any way you can as long as you don't get caught even if it's against the law; or, one can engage in unethical behaviors until they are outlawed, the old "buyer beware".

This unethical conscience that I am speaking of manifests as collusion with the injustices of society that seem to affect others but most people also overlook the injustices that affect everyone in the society. Really deep down, not everyone, but most people are okay with those ideas of survival of the fittest, buyer beware, etc. Most ordinary people feel it is alright for certain individuals to get "filthy rich", etc. while others, even themselves, linger in economic distress because they somehow think that maybe they might win the lottery or maybe they too might be able to be someone in power, one of the rich and famous. Agreeing with this ideal, most people accept higher crime by ordinary criminals as well as politicians and corporations, and allow disparities in the justice system, disparities in income and other injustices, thinking that these are necessary in order to have a society where it is possible to become "filthy rich."

There are men, however, who though they do not belong to the privileged order, say they like it, because it affords every man at least a chance of becoming a nobleman.

The United States magazine and Democratic review, Volume 6, 1839 C.E.

This syndrome in the population of the countries that have an economy controlled by the rich through credit, was recognized as early as the year 1839. Anyone wishing to understand the purpose and workings of the pseudo–capitalist credit based banking system of the western countries and how it operates for the benefit of the rich and how it systematically impoverishes the rest of the population while deceiving the masses, should read *The United States magazine and Democratic review*, Volume 6, 1839 C.E.

*Nothing can be more demoralizing than our
bank-nobility system. "Give me neither
poverty nor riches," was the prayer of
Augur, "lest I be full, and deny thee, and
say, Who is the Lord? Or lest I be poor, and
steal, and take the nance of my God in
vain." As the whole operation of our
banking-system is to enrich one class of men
by impoverishing another, it would e
difficult to devise a more efficient means of
destroying that happy mediocrity of fortune
which is so favorable to the practice of
Christian and republican values.*
**The United States magazine and Democratic
review, Volume 6, 1839 C.E.**

So, on that basis, it's okay for others to be
controlled or to be stepped on or even themselves to
be stepped on a little. It's a very interesting
negative psychological condition. That's not the
only one; there's a kind of mixed pathology in
many people's minds where they accept the feeling
that they're slaves, or at least subservient and
impotent. Many people do not think that they're
worthy to be anything but a follower, a consumer,
and do whatever they are told since they have been
convinced that their country can do no wrong and
their leaders are there because they are most able,
and or that the system is to big and cannot be
changed by anything they do, etc. Others are fearful
of change while still others are fearful of what they
consider to be the "evil government", that the
government may put laws upon them that will hurt
them. These are the kinds of people that are misled
by those in positions of power to promote less

government regulations so that they, the wealthy, may operate in a lawless environment and thereby be able to take advantage of the majority, the people who are made to feel fear about losing their freedoms.

In a sense it's a schizophrenic culture. That is, it's a disease whereby people are conditioned to voting for things that are detrimental to themselves and following ignorance instead of reason as well as following the greedy who they are told have their (the masses) welfare at heart, their well-being at heart, but in reality it's about money and power; that is, taking wealth from the masses and maintaining them in their place through policing, and the legal, penal and economic systems that the elite can afford to finance and therefore, direct. This of course, is a boon for the power elite because they do not need to impose their will by force since they have fostered a society full of ignorant gullible serfs, thinking they have free will, not realizing they are enslaved by bankers through credit and meager wages. This new development in history, of a society bamboozled, not requiring subjugation by force, but by indoctrination and deception by the wealthy, and the dangers to society, was written about in the early 19th century and more recently extensively explored and defined by researchers such as Michael Parenti[21] and Noam Chomsky in his presentation called *Manufacturing Consent.*[22]

---

[21] *Inventing Reality: The Politics of the Mass Media* by Michael Parenti (Paperback - 1986)
[22] *Manufacturing Consent: The Political Economy of the Mass Media* (1988), by Edward S. Herman and Noam Chomsky,

The problem of the power elite (nobility) has been known about since early in the history of the USA.

> *"The nobility systems of other countries having been established by force, and being supported by force, can perhaps be got rid of only by force. But our American nobility system being founded in fraud and supported by fraud, can be got rid of in no other way than by effectually exposing the nature of that fraud."*
> **The United States magazine and Democratic review, Volume 6, 1839 C.E.**

Those same ordinary ignorant people, the masses (poor and middle class) are willing to serve the rich and powerful thinking they have a chance to someday be like them. They have been convinced that the rich and powerful, who were, in an earlier period, referred to as the nobility, the aristocrats, know best and in their benevolence will create decent jobs for everyone. We have seen throughout history that the power elite do not share their wealth benevolently but by necessity only; otherwise they hoard their wealth and employ it to control government so as not to lose wealth and power and even to have laws in their favor so that they might increase it.

So the masses, through their ignorance and greed, are complicit in their own miserable predicament. In this sense they are not unlike marks that have become victims of con artists, swindlers; but here we see the con job has been and continues to be massive and society wide. They achieve neither socio/economic fairness nor good government because their own corruption causes them to follow the wealthy and allow them to stay in power.

And that is not what we had in ancient Kemet. I wanted to go over some proverbs and teachings from the wisdom text sages who discussed the higher principles that a society should be governed by and the ethical principles that a human being, even in business, in commerce, should be guided by. So these teachings apply to all socio-economic classes of the society.

The wisdom texts are a particular genre of Ancient Egyptian literature often characterized as didactic since it provides specific instructions on proper understanding of life, the proper behavior in relationships with other humans and with the earth and the proper treatment of human beings and of nature. There are some main genres of texts of ancient Kemet that form what we call the ancient writings or ancient scriptures. The proper African/Ancient Egyptian name for them is *Medtu Neter*. Some of them are writings that were related to the nature of the afterlife, the Netherworld, and the original ones or the earliest ones of those are referred to as Pyramid Texts. The next developments in that genre were the Coffin Texts and the final development of that genre was called the Book of the Dead or the Pert em Hru text.

The first ones were written in stone; the second were written in wood; and the third were written on papyri. Then you have the genre of text known as wisdom texts; these are kinds of teachings that are didactic writings of the sages, those who are recognized as sages of the early phase of Ancient

Egyptian history. In a sense they laid the groundwork or a foundation for the Ma'atian teachings, the philosophy that we call Ma'at which is really a foundation for the entire social order of ancient Kemet.

Maat Philosophy is what allowed them to have a well ordered and prosperous society for thousands of years. This philosophy is the seed, this is the DNA upon which the societal philosophy of Ancient Egypt was based, what allowed them to have a culture existing in harmony with itself and with nature for thousands of years as opposed to what we see now in the United States, a culture that after a mere 234 years is so schizophrenic that it is tearing itself apart politically and economically as well as tearing up the environment and damaging or destroying other cultures through war or economic subjugation and exploitation.[23]

"If the social order judges success by material gain, the most successful will be the most corruptible and selfish."
-Ancient Egyptian Proverb

So the wisdom texts are a particular genre of teachings given by individual sages, referencing the philosophy that a human being should live by in order to be in harmony with nature and in harmony with the universe and in so doing being in harmony with spirit, with the divine, with God, which is the overall goal of life, to be one with the Supreme and transcending one's human limitations in order to

---

[23] See the book: *Collapse of Civilization* by Muata Ashby

discover one's higher self and to be all that one truly can be.

Did they come before the Pyramid Texts and Coffin Texts or they came after that with the foundation for the Ma'atian teachings that you just described?

Muata Ashby: That's a good question. The earliest of the wisdom texts that have come down to us, which have survived through history, are from the Old Kingdom period and some of them actually have been lost to history or they have not been discovered yet. It's very likely they are under the sands of Kemet, like the writings from sages such as Imhotep. So the earliest come from the period when the early afterlife texts were also being written.

Imhotep was an architect, lawyer, a doctor, a philosopher, a true genius of his time and he was known to have certain writings that have not been discovered yet but history talks about them. And there are others who are well known like Ptahotep who wrote some of the earliest wisdom texts.

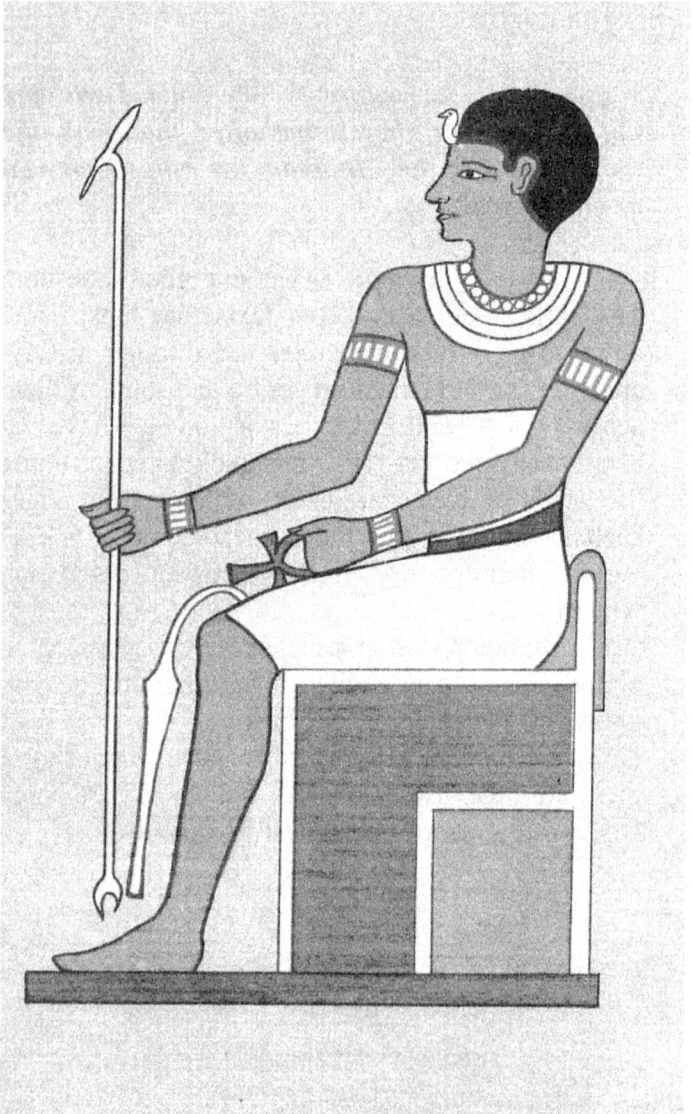

Figure 14: Ancient Egyptian sage Imhotep

Let's start with forgiveness of debts. One of the teachings states that if a man can't pay his debt, one should forgive two-thirds of the debt and hold him or her responsible for one third. This method constitutes ethical disposition of debt, unlike this culture (U.S.A.) which actually has really turned negative towards the disposition of debt in the sense that many people are not aware that just a few years ago, about five years ago, a bankruptcy law came into being, whereby people are not forgiven their debts anymore. This allows corporations to go after them even after they have nothing.

In prior years, the bankruptcy law for corporations and for individuals, allowed the debts of those who were deemed to be qualified to file for bankruptcy, to wash away their debts so they could start over; to start over without the burden. But now they (those in control) don't want that. Now they are going to try to take everything you have and then leave you in debt so that you'll be basically in slavery, perpetual indentured servitude kind of slavery. You'll have to work for repaying your debts and you'll never really be able to start over.

Now the problem is worse because of the new law that came into being by the rich corporations buying off the congress. The law now allows them to take most of a person's property and once the bankruptcy goes through, the bankrupt person is required to pay 25 percent of their income towards the debt but the creditor now can also charge 30 percent interest. So the bankrupt person can actually end up owing more than the original debt and it is also possible that they will never be free of the burden of the debt. But what is the alternative to such a system? This is a prime example of how the credit based economic system is used to maintain people in perpetual debt and thus beholding to those in control. This is how a banking system is setup to financially enslave a population for the profit of the bank's owners. In contrast, if a bank were to be setup as a utility, like an electric utility, or water and sewer utility, to service an entire community, not controlled by individuals for profit, but rather, administered by the government for the purpose of providing needed funds, as a public service, for development and benefit of all members of the society then there would be no development of debt slaves and no capacity for the rich, the nobility, to form cabals to control the economy or impoverish the masses while creating extreme imbalances between the wealth of the masses and the wealth of the few rich. Such banking systems exist today and where they do exist there have been no swindles by the bankers, no loss of State revenues due to banking malfeasance, no extraction of wealth from the population, no real estate crises due to the banking malpractice and or corruption, no undermining of stock markets, no crashes of the economy, etc. Such an example is the banking system of the State of North Dakota.

> As the only state-owned bank in the nation, our mission, established by legislative action in 1919, is to promote agriculture, commerce and industry in North Dakota. The Bank acts as a

funding resource in partnership with other financial institutions, economic development groups and guaranty agencies. We have four established business areas: Student Loans, Lending Services, Treasury Services and Banking Services.[24]

This is the same kind of process as the prison industrial complex as it is a mechanism of keeping people in the penal system, keeping them from being able to vote or keeping them from being able to gain and accumulate wealth that would provide the chance to have the capacity to forge their own destiny. The banking system, the prison industrial complex, and many other aspects of the society are socio-economic-political mechanisms establishing and maintaining a process of impoverishing people and maintaining them powerless. These are forms of institutionalized corruption in the society.

The teaching is that if one were to be able to apply righteous and ethical practices in finances as well as in spiritual life, one would be able to be free physically and mentally from the negative or the inimical forces of the world be those forces in the form of people trying to enslave a person physically with chains or enslave them with debt, with a mortgage or whatever else it may be. That is the external enslavement. A person also needs to seek freedom from their own fears and unethical desires. It is those internal unethical desires, the slavery to one's own unethical desires, which leads to the external slavery.

---

[24] http://www.banknd.nd.gov/

So, ultimately, people are also enslaving themselves with illusions about life - I have to have a big house, I have to have three cars, I have to have several children, I have to have whatever I think I have to have. That is the problem that is going to trap you, especially in the times that we're living in now.

So I'd like to go through this next one, which is a teaching that relates to business and commerce and it comes from Sage Amenemope. This comes from the proverbs, *"those who give away their treasure wisely give away their plagues. They that retain their increase heap up sorrow."* This teaching gives the idea of the irony of rich people. The question is asked: "how much is enough" and then the answer is "it's never enough." People, who are rich, are no different from the poor in that they too upset and agitation regardless of their wealth. In some ways it is worse for them because they can to some extent shield themselves with their money and distract themselves with possessions, travel and other activities and not face the harshness of life, as those with less wealth may have to. Through that confrontation they might have developed humility and dispassion about the world of illusion leading to real peace and contentment in life.

After one million, two million, 10 million. How many millions are enough? In a sense, part of this pathology is created or caused by fear. Many of the same people who get rich, since they know it is an ill-gotten gain, or due to general insecurity due to their knowledge of the corrupt economic system that is designed to take wealth from the masses and transfer it to the top 1% of the population, the super rich; they're afraid they might lose it too, so they think that no amount is sufficient because it can be lost at any given point due to the government and economic system setup, due to an accident, theft, or maybe the poor and or minorities may finally wise up and revolt, etc. So the insecurity fostered by the unethical system of economics and government, feeds the desire to get more and more, even if it is at the expense of others or at the expense of ones own physical or mental health or at the expense of ones own ethics, i.e. crime. If you have a lopsided culture where people can become so fabulously rich, it means that other people have to become fabulously impoverished. That means it's an ill-gotten gain in that sense, generally. It is fundamentally unfair to have such an imbalance in the distribution of wealth.

> The misery our system inflicts on the commonality is indescribable and yet it imparts but a comparatively small degree of happiness to the nobility. Their fortunes are as unsteady as the stock market. This they know and feel, and even in the midst of their most splendid revelries, a cloud creeps over their brow from a lurking sense of the danger that attends them…the nobles are not content because they know not how soon they will be reduced to poverty, and we, the common people, are not content, because we all want to become *ricos hombres,* or nobles.
>
> The United States magazine and Democratic review, Volume 6, 1839 C.E.

The fear of loss is a deep seated fear in the hearts of most members of the society but especially in those who have achieved inordinate wealth. It is a fear that contributes to the population's acquiescence to what amount to criminal acts by politicians and corporate leaders who say they are acting to protect the "American way of life" or "protecting the interests of the USA," or as they label those government leaders that resist American Imperial hegemony as communists, dictators, or now the worst, terrorists. This is a way to demonize them and facilitate the use of force to replace them with truly corrupt leaders that will favor the policies of American multinational corporation's needs for raw materials and or populations that will work for slave level wages. So the rich are fearful that they're going to lose their wealth and so they think, well, the best way to ensure myself is to get more, as much as they can, without any end. And this, of course, leads a human being to stress and to disease as well as insanity. So these are the great ills or plagues that wealth can bring if the mind is caught up in fear and greed, degradation conscience and egoism. But a society does not have to live by fear to have prosperity; the Ancient Egyptian society demonstrated that by instituting laws and financial policies that were designed to harness the benefits of cooperation and fair distribution of resources.

It also means that wealth is a kind of tool which should be deployed in the form of righteous investments and it should not be hoarded because the more it is hoarded the more it denies the human community of its benefits. Wealth can become a disease like the accumulation in the body, of toxins and distorted cells that are going to cause cancer and death.

So one who achieves wealth then should endeavor to give it away? Is that what we're being instructed and taught from the ancient sages and saints?

Muata Ashby: Essentially yes, but not exactly as one might think. We are really talking about sharing, maintaining fair and proper allocation of resources in a society to maintain order, peace and justice. The Ma'atian philosophy is not an extreme so it doesn't mean that you give everything away and leave yourself with nothing. From a practical standpoint everyone needs some amount of wealth to sustain their day to day activities. Yet, it means that you use what is necessary for your survival, for your own work that you do and to maintain the legitimate needs of life or for education or other righteous endeavors, then the excess that is not needed is to be put to a good use and that could be a good investment in some kind of building, a project or process that improves the community. It could be many different things, it could be helping others, or helping family, giving to community projects or charitable projects and it can also be community service in the form of volunteering to help others but also contributions in art, philosophy, science, etc. When we are talking about charity we are not talking about charity in a sense that most people may think about that today; we are not referring to philanthropy in a modern day sense.

Think about it, if we had a cooperative society where everyone contributes to the well-being of everyone else we would have universal healthcare, housing and work opportunities for all. Then people would not need to feel insecure about their finances. We have a lopsided society with fabulously rich people on one side and everyone else on the other. We are not talking about philanthropy in the sense of charity where the richer folk get to give handouts to the poorer folk and get deductions on their taxes and get to delude themselves thinking they have done good for society. We're talking about real altruism, temple building and opportunity for all and not just for the few. Kemetic economics should be thought of in a higher context and not in the context that we think of for present day culture, what this culture calls charity and philanthropy.

How should wealth be used in those types of endeavors, how is that helpful to society and the individual?

Muata Ashby: Well, consider that current society, modern society, would not necessarily see this philosophy as something beneficial. We can look on the twin towers (World Trade Center) that fell when the attack was made on them in 2001, as the pillars and monuments to wealth and greed of this country. What can we say that that accumulation of wealth, represented by the towers, brought forth? It brought forth the fear and condemnation, anger and aggression of other cultures because in gaining that wealth this country had to and continues to damage or destroy other cultures and it had to destroy other people's governments and economies, like the ones in South America, Africa, the Middle East and other places. How did the USA become the most powerful country in the world? It has had a long history of undermining the governments and economies and attacking other countries to prevent them from gaining wealth and protecting their wealth (in the form of natural resources) from USA corporations and preventing them from being competitive with western economies. Several European countries are complicit in this process as well. That is how the United States (wealthy in control of the banks and cabal industries mentioned earlier) gained wealth, by preventing others and by enslaving others, not to mention the massacring of the Native Americans and the theft of their lands.[25]

If we were to create temples or monuments, to the divine, as opposed to greed but more than just to the divine, to a philosophy of truth, a philosophy of righteousness and order, caring and fairness, then we would have the kind of wealth that the Ancient Egyptians had, the wealth of prosperity, the wealth of long life, not just as individuals but as a society. Additionally, Ancient Egyptian Maat philosophy, as the foundation for commerce, economics and government promoted the principle of care for the

---

[25] See the book: *Collapse of Civilization* by Muata Ashby

environment. Ancient Egyptian society existed for thousands of years through preservation of the environment. We see what's happening with this culture; its depleting it's own natural resources and those of the entire world. This culture is not balanced as the Ancient Egyptian but instead it is founded in a culture of greed and excess.

It's not only depleting its natural resources, it's depleting its human resources, and it's depleting its human wits, its nerves. The culture of the USA and other countries founded in the same principles, are living in constant fear and economic stress which leads to discontentment and animosity; notice the high unemployment, the high murder rate and high incarceration rate, higher than all other supposedly developed countries; This points not to development in the direction of civilization, what Ancient Egypt hand, but rather development in the direction of barbarism, of feudalism. I think that the wealth that is balanced, sustainable, renewable and thus perennial, the wealth that transcends from generation to generation, that is true wealth, as opposed to the wealth that uses up people, the wealth that burdens people, that transfers from the general public to a small minority of greedy, scared, sociopathic or pathological individuals. So these are the teachings of wealth of Ancient Kemet, the higher order of wealth as opposed to what people call wealth now which is essentially material wealth and wealth that is fleeting, wealth that really cannot bring happiness.

I mean, it causes stress and sorrow. There's material wealth that can bring a certain amount of stability and a certain amount of wealth is necessary to have a life but that need not be such that it causes imbalances between haves and have nots. Last time we discussed the three Maatian responsibilities designed to meet the three main needs of a human being - the need for food and for shelter and for opportunity. Beyond that, material wealth is not really helpful to discovering abiding happiness and abiding contentment. For that, it's necessary to have a different kind of perspective, a different kind of study whereby a person is able to discover the meaning of life and has the opportunity to work towards fulfilling, and indeed realizing that meaning in the form of a purposeful and rewarding, contented professional and spiritual life. For that purpose, the ancients devised the science of Shetaut Neter (Egyptian Mysteries) and Sema Tawi (Egyptian Yoga), and Maat philosophy (Ethical and balanced way of life).[26]

It is important to note that we are discussing the highest ideal of Ancient Egyptian philosophy. Its practice was reduced in the late period of Ancient Egyptian history when barbarians such as the Assyrians, Persians, Greeks and Romans attacked and finally conquered Egypt. It is important for everyone to realize that the Hollywood depictions of ancient Egypt have no basis in reality and many of the portrayals in documentaries, like those on the History Channel and Learning Channel, are also equally flawed in various ways. It's important to note that the later period that was known as the late period of Ancient

---

[26] www.egyptianyoga.com/catalog

Egyptian history, which is somewhere after 600 or 700 BCE, that period is a period of much turmoil in which the Persians, Assyrians, Romans, the Greeks all tried to conquer and some succeeded in conquering Egypt for a period of time until the Greeks finally conquered it for good. Many aspects of the culture were distorted, corrupted, stopped or otherwise changed by those outside cultures that came in. So, indeed, many of the beliefs or traditions that have been advertised as being Ancient Egyptian were not so; therefore, it's important to have that distinction when engaging in Ancient Egyptian studies.

Let's look at the next proverb that provides insights into the nature of economics and financial affairs. *"Help your friends with the things that you have for you have these things by the grace of God. If you fail to help your friends, one will say you have a selfish soul. One plans for tomorrow but you do not know what tomorrow will bring. The right soul is the soul by which one is sustained. If you do praise-worthy deeds your friends will say welcome in your time of need."*

Many people think about the architecture and iconography of Ancient Egypt but do not think of Ancient Egyptian culture and the philosophy it is founded upon. This is a culture that existed before the Greeks, the Romans, before the Arabs, before the Persians came in. This is essentially an African culture, founded by African people who had migrated to Ancient Kemet (Egypt) from the area that is today called Uganda and Sudan which was also known previously as Nubia and Kush. And as such, they followed the fundamental principles of African ethics, and culture. I discussed this topic in a book called *Matrix of African Proverbs*.

And one of the most important principles is of community. It is a "we" oriented culture as opposed to a "me" oriented culture. In this current western culture, everything is about me, you know, you gain your wealth and other people gain their wealth and supposedly everything is supposed to work well while other people are competing to gain wealth but somebody has to lose. It's a zero sum game the way it's played in this culture; in order for some to gain others must lose. But it does not have to be a zero sum game; it is that way because those in power have chosen things to be that way. People of a different cultural viewpoint can choose a different way, and many have even today. Just as in Ancient Egypt, some countries today have chosen to take care of all members of the society in varied ways, such as with healthcare for all and not allow people to fend for themselves in a world where some people have different capacities than others.

There needs to be a shift to the understanding that we are all better off if there is fair sharing of resources rather than allowing the few to enjoy and control most off the resources. This also means accepting the idea that we are all related in spirit and also related in genetics. All human beings are related genetically. All human beings are kinfolks in essence and there's no such thing as races - races of white people, black people, yellow people, whatever. And since human beings exist in and depend on a social world and social relationships; no human being can exist as an individual from the time that they are born, they rightly and appropriately join with others to have support and to work towards a common goal to promote proper availability of needed resources for survival and finally, create optimal conditions for attaining spiritual enlightenment. That's what society is supposed to be there for.

And if you contribute to society, if you help others, others will be very willing and able to help you in your time of need. And that is one of the main benefits of family, main benefits of society, and those who break that trust, those who seek wealth without restriction, without ethics, being wealthy while other people are languishing in disease or languishing in poverty, this is immoral and is obscene. And this kind of activity tears society apart and it robs a society from its core, eating away at people's ethical conscience, which is what this current culture has been doing virtually from its inception. And that is what this proverb is relating to.

I think the ideal of the texts speaks of the family of humanity as a whole. So the application of this idea, of this teaching as related in our current condition, would be as follows. For example, those people who have been harmed by the bankers who created the real estate bubble of the years 2001-2008, the bankers who knowingly made loans to them that they should not have made and who also forged documents so they could get these people to sign up for loans and so they (bankers and others) could get the benefits of commissions those loans and then later foreclosing on the properties for even more profits, the victims should be free of debt and the bankers should take the losses of their own malfeasance and fraud and be fined and jailed.

The people, who were or are facing or are in foreclosure, should be helped. They should not lose their property. The bankers and others, who caused the situation, should be the ones going to jail, that should be punished, whose wealth should be confiscated to pay the damages of what they have done and they should not be rewarded or bailed out; that would be the mark of a real step towards fixing the economic malfeasance and corruption of the culture. But we see that is not happening. Those people are being even rewarded with more wealth. People in Congress who allowed the unrighteousness are being rewarded with more wealth as well.

When they get out of congress they're hired by the same people who perpetrated this crime. So they are paid off before, during and after their time in congress. This is the sustenance of the corruption in government, legalized bribes (campaign contributions) which the rich are most capable of offering to those who do their bidding. A person who is highly ethical in this sense will not be sitting idle or would not be insensitive to the issues or problems of people even if they're across the world because it is really one human family in that sense.

This next proverb I'll go through is coming to the idea of some aspects of personal finances as well as finances in business. This is by Sage Ani.

"The wealth accrues to him who guards it; let your hand not scatter it to strangers, lest it turn to loss for you. If wealth is placed where there is interest, it comes back to you redoubled. Make a storehouse for your own wealth, your people will find it on your way. What is given small returns augmented, what is replaced brings abundance."

This teaching by Sage Ani is essentially about how to make wealth, how to make proper investments; he's talking about not squandering and giving out lightly to strangers or to people like con artists or people who come with ideas that haven't been well thought out and he does not make a distinction between strangers or family members. The focus here is on truth, what is viable, as well as who is the investment with, how well are they known, what is the reputation and the track record to support a future prospect that would be beneficial and positive?

This is the notion of being thoughtful, of placing your funds, your wealth where it will be secure and employed prudently, where it will properly grow as an investment. Before entering into an investment one should thoroughly check out the person or institution the investment will be with, making sure they are reputable, in order to avoid losses as much as possible. And these principles are not taught to people. When I was growing up in high school, there were classes of Home Economics and subjects like that. and we see how, especially since the '80s, since the Ronald Reagan, Republicans came into power, many of those basic classes that were in high schools before have been taken out and replaced with really inane subjects, subjects that help people to be better followers and better slaves as opposed to classes and subjects that help people to be able to think for themselves and to make better decisions based on facts and common sense beyond egoism and greed or religious fundamentalism based on blind faith.

This issue is especially highlighted as we see that in the elementary and secondary curriculums of some states like Texas the school boards are even rewriting the history in the books to take certain things out of history that they don't want people, especially young people, to know; this is state sponsored and institutionalized miseducation. This is not a way of creating a society of strong people who have individual conscience and also ethical societal conscience. It is a way of creating masses of ignorant slaves. So this kind of teaching, such as the Ancient Egyptian Maat, if it were applied by those who are poor or powerless, not squandering their money and giving it away to Hollywood entertainments, buying tickets to go see *American Idol* or football games or for cigarettes, expensive and unnecessary hair weaves, or to follow corrupt politicians, then those funds could be better invested and one could eventually have a wealthy life.

We've been talking mostly about material abundance but the same principles apply to spiritual abundance as well. People squander vast amounts of wealth at churches, Mosques, etc that may give them a temporary feeling of spiritual relief or sense of community where everybody is jumping up and down, screaming hallelujah or bowing repeatedly in a reverential manner producing a feeling of devotion but since it is based on faith only, faith that does not require ethical conscience[27], it doesn't give them true spiritual wealth, the kind of wealth that you can take with you and live a strong, independent life and even be a pillar for society, the kind of wealth that is a foundation for societal peace and harmony and ultimately higher spiritual awakenings. It is, rather, a kind of enslavement, both physical and psychological as well as financial. That is what you get from most of the faith-based churches and mosques. One may think that mega churches are good because they have thousands of members and may give thousands in donations but their pastors never speak out against government corruption or the sinful ways of their members who are corporate leaders who specialize in taking advantage of the masses in their own country and abroad as well. So the priests, ministers, pastors, Rabbis, Imams of orthodox religions are complicit in the malfeasance, and general corruptions of the politicians they support, who in turn support them, as well as the system of government and economics

---

[27] Faith-based religion does not require ethical conscience of their followers, only faith; transgressions can be forgiven, so ethics are not a requirement. Ex. Churches in the USA have not spoken out against American imperialism, the disparity of wealth, etc. Churches, Mosques and Synagogues are facilitators to the unrighteous actions of Plutocracy and fascism. See the book *Limits of Faith* by Muata Ashby

which is fundamentally unfair and corrupt. So this proverb really has many ramifications.

This particular teaching is not only referring to the personal wealth but it definitely applies in the same way to the communal wealth. Think of how, once you're able to accumulate wealth, you can assist others, help others, and be of benefit to others. That applies also to the wealth of knowledge; it applies to the wealth of spiritual evolution, of spiritual self-discovery, things that you can share with others, things that you can give to others that money really cannot give.

The next teaching comes from Sage Ankhsheshonq, *"Do not lend money at interest without obtaining a security and do not be too trusting lest you become poor."* Consider that these teachings are from a period before the western banks came into being. This recalls the ideal of being prudent, not giving money to charlatans, spin doctors or con artists, or people who knock on your door trying to sell you something or people on TV or politicians or anyone for that matter, people trying to sell you, sell even themselves as someone likable or trustworthy but who are in reality charlatans preying on your ignorance and or other incapacities.

The concept of security really has more dimensions than just physical money. But looking at the mundane aspects of this, in reference to giving money, one should not give money that one is not comfortable with losing because there is always some risk and that means that you have to see what is affordable since it makes no sense to invest with such risk as to cause oneself ruin if the investment goes negatively. This concept applies to lending money to relatives also; what purpose would it serve to lend money to a relative and then you end up poor as well? What purpose does it serve that both instead of one will be out of a house to live in or have to give up a car, etc.? Better to calculate what you can afford to lose (the amount you can lend and still be OK if it never comes back) without jeopardizing the wealth you need to sustain your basic expenses and then lend that amount. It is important to maintain one's financial base and work with disposable capital. This policy also helps in being able to make investment decisions without undue stress from worrying about the fate of the investment due to having to rely on it for one's fundamental expenses of life. So, of course you should try to take a security, collateral, if we're speaking in the context of a business or even in personal matters. Consider that if you are prudent with your finances you can be more serviceable to others. If one falls on hard times it would not be prudent for you to give what you have and also end up in hard times with them; better to retain your capacities so you can be of better assistance. For example, if a person loses their job and their house is foreclosed do not lend them money just to extend their time in the house if there are no prospects to get a job that can sustain the house in the future. Better to let them lose the house and save your money. You can offer them to live with you until they get back on their feet and the funds you saved can be used to sustain any added expenses due to having the new guests. You cannot save everyone and should not extend a helping hand blindly, without wise contemplation before you take action. One more thing about this, one should not allow oneself to overlook the truth; the truth is not related to who is a friend, a compatriot, a member of one's social group or political party, family or "race" etc. Also, your decisions should not be based on guilt, say if you feel bad because you did not lend money the last time so you feel you should lend it now regardless, or because it is a family member, etc. Is this truth? This is the important question. Does the loan have a basis in truth or is it illusory? Answer this first and then see if the economics are there to make the loan possible and prudent. Remember that other people have their own ariu they need to work through. To some extent you can be a mitigating factor for them but if you transgress beyond the bounds of propriety you will be doing them and yourself a disservice and potentially hurt theirs and your capacity for spiritual evolution, creating more physical, mental and spiritual bonds to the world of illusion by creating more attachments, anxieties and unnecessary toils by now having to overcome the new debt burdens. In the end your considerations cannot be in contradiction with truth and all other considerations are secondary. Any of those groups can have con artists and any in those groups can make mistakes in their calculations and not be able to pay or they may die unexpectedly, all because their *ariu* decreed it. One should not fall into the trap either of sentimentality or of familiarity; this is not callousness because you do care and you will not leave them without some assistance, if possible, but you also must uphold your principles too. Actually, if you apply these principles you will be helping them in the best way possible. Do not be compromised by sentimentalities that force you to overlook truth. Be consistent in your application of this standard and others may not like it but they will understand and respect it.

But thinking that if one is going to be righteous in lending, which means being a bank in a sense, then the chances of that loan going into foreclosure or arrears should be minimized because you're doing it with a righteous context and not like what has been done with the mortgages in this country (USA) where people were given loans that the banks knew they could not afford, even expecting them to fail so they could make money on commissions from the initial loan and then come back and take the property on foreclosure and make even more money by selling it at auction; so that whole process was unrighteous there from the start and is still. Thus, there is a prudent way of practicing lending and borrowing.

The next teaching reads: *"borrow money at interest and put it in farmlands. Borrow money at interest and take a wife. Borrow money at interest and celebrate your birthday. Do not borrow money at interest in order to live well on earth."* The last line is really the key. There are many things that one can borrow money for if one is going to invest. It is okay to borrow money if it is within a righteous amount of interest and the right features to the loan and if it is for the right purpose.

A loan should not be of a usurious kind that will keep you enslaved, paying more in interest than the original principle, causing years of payments and depleting resources from better uses. You can borrow money to invest in things that gain in value, to get married, to found a house, to have a foundation for your home, start a business, or for onetime event needs and things like that. But you should not borrow money to live on, for vacations, frivolous entertainments, etc. These are not proper investments, since they do not appreciate in value; rather, they will squander the wealth. So, in the wrong investments a person will end up essentially expending or exhausting, in other words: "squandering" the wealth and not having the future benefits the wealth could have brought through growth and appreciation. If it was invested properly you could have had the wealth and the comfort of living well. These are prudent actions that a person should take for their personal finances.

We will conclude this section with the teaching of Sage Amenemope on the prayer for wealth. Let's read a few lines and then we'll end with a prayer for wealth.

"Do not set your heart on wealth. There is no ignoring fate and destiny. Do not let your heart go straying; every man comes to his hour. Do not strain to seek increase. What you have, let it suffice you. If riches come to you by theft, they will not stay the night with you. Come day they are not in your house. Their place is seen

but they are not there. Do not rejoice in wealth from theft, nor complain of being poor. If the leading archer presses forward, his company abandons him; the boat of the greedy is left in the mud, while the bark of the silent sails with the wind. Get into the habit of praying sincerely to Aton as he rises in the sky, saying grant me strength, well-being and health (di a sekhem, udja, senab). He will give you your needs for this life and you will be safe from fear."

Most people pray to win a lottery ticket or to do well in business or get a promotion. That is the destiny they want but they ignore the idea of *ariu*. In our terms, this means, the sum total of your previous deeds, your feelings, your desires and experiences that has an effect on what you feel and think now and thus what you will do in the future or what your fate will be in the future. This means that you can want something consciously but your basis of feeling and desiring from the past may work against the present desires. This manifests as people striving but failing through no apparent fault of their own or people failing due to sabotaging their own efforts towards what they say they want. So you should not pray to be wealthy or to be rich and you should not be looking forward to or be afraid of being poor.

You need to live a balanced life and direct yourself towards righteousness and truth and everything necessary and beneficial will be achieved from there. In the Kemetic Medtu Neter (hieroglyphic text), the saying, grant me strength, well-being and health translates to *di a sekhem, udja, senab*. This is the prayer, strength, well-being and health. That will bring all the wealth and all the health that is necessary for life.

PART 3:
QUESTIONS AND
ANSWERS

Wealth may be considered as one's physical, mental and or spiritual capacity to pursue and sustain well-being and the capacity to pursue spiritual enlightenment.

-Sebai Dr. Muata Ashby

Question: How does Kemetic Economics apply to the current conditions of the United States and world economy today?

Answer

Udja (Greetings)
These are critically important questions for our times. As a follower of Shetaut Neter, meaning for those initiated at Shems or Asar levels it is important to apply the principles of Kemetic economics that I have discussed in several lectures; primarily there must be prudence in dealing with expenses, taking or offering loans and when investing. If these principles are followed they constitute a foundation for one's own life, to meet one's financial needs. I think the following Ancient Egyptian proverbs hold important teachings for today.

> *The one who has wealth at home will not be partial;*
> *He is a just man who lacks nothing.*
> *The poor man does not speak justly,*
> *Not righteous is one, who says, "I wish I had,"*
> **-Ancient Egyptian Sage MeriKaRa**

(41) "I have never magnified my condition beyond what was fitting or increased my wealth, except with such things as are (justly) mine own possessions by means of Maat." <u>Variant: I have not disputed over possessions except when they concern my own rightful possessions. Variant: I have not desired more than what is rightfully mine.</u>

**--from the Ancient Egyptian
42 Precepts of Maat**

A healthy society needs to have balance in the wealth of its citizens. *"The one who has wealth at home will not be partial..."* means, not that the more rich people there are the more justice and fairness those people will be, for we see in present day society exactly the opposite, they are more greedy, selfish and criminal. Rather, it means that when people feel secure in the basics of life they will not act with partiality, with partisanship, not caring about the needs or fate of others. A society that promotes a healthy balance in the differences of wealth of the members of the society necessarily needs to be ethical and prudent in the distribution of the resources of the society. This means being ethical in personal as well as business dealings but prudence means wise ethics; you should not give a loan to a person you know is unrighteous, who will squander it and later give some inane excuse for not being able to pay it back. Likewise you should not take a loan that seeks to enslave you with usurious interest. Money may be thought of as a form of potential energy and as a tool that can be used for righteousness or unrighteousness. When you use moneys either from your labor, your business or from loans that is to be invested wisely, first in legitimate expenses of living, *Ra-the Sustainer,* to maintain a household, etc. and not squandered in non-necessities. A portion is held in reserve (held as savings or as commodities-gold, real estate, seeds, food, etc.) for eventuality or when needed, *Amun-the Observer,* and another portion is then put to work in conservative wise investments, *Ptah-the Creation.*

...wealth does not come by itself.
-Ancient Egyptian Sage Ptahotep

Wealth may be considered as one's physical, mental and or spiritual capacity to pursue and sustain well-being and the capacity to pursue spiritual enlightenment. One may have lots of physical wealth (money, cars, and houses) but at the same time have also mental anguish, unrest, sorrow. One may have lots of money and at the same time also spiritual bankruptcy; a person can be rich but at the same time can also be empty or evil. Physical wealth does not automatically bring mental or spiritual wealth but it is a foundation to allow a person to pursue mental and spiritual fulfillment. So physical wealth in the form of moneys, and things that can be equated with monetary value (real estate, food, car, computer, etc.), is an important and legitimate consideration when determining one's physical needs and mental and spiritual desires for peace and contentment. The amount of physical wealth needed is determined by the economy one lives in. Therefore one person may live in a society where most things are expensive while another may live in a country or culture where things are much simpler and the cost of living is lower. The cost of living is an important determiner of the amount of effort needed to sustain a basic lifestyle (a lifestyle that sustains the basic needs of life (food/water, clothing, shelter, opportunity). In fairer, more ethical countries, the cost of living is fairer while in pseudo-capitalist societies, the cost of living is inordinately higher. Of course there are many other factors to consider like the level of income, one's job or career, etc. the important thing to remember is that when an economy is in balance a person is able to live reasonably well without undue stress; they are able to live off wages and be able to sustain the main needs of life, food, shelter and opportunity. If a society does not allow a person to achieve these basic needs, without undue stress and strife, it is out of balance.

> (23) The beggar in God's hand is better off than the rich man in his palace.
> Crusts of bread and a loving heart are better than rich food and mental agitation.
> Hanker therefore after daintiness.
> Mind thy business, and let every man do his when he wishes to do it.
> Learn to be content with what thou hast.

(24) Better is poverty in the hand of
The God, Than -wealth in the
storehouse;
Better is bread with a happy heart,
Than wealth with vexation.

**-Ancient Egyptian Sage
Amenemope**

Do not rely on another's goods
(possessions),
Guard what you acquire yourself;
Do not depend on another's wealth,
Lest he become master in your
house.
Build a house or find and buy one,
Shun contention
Don't say: "My mother's father has a
house,
'A house that lasts,' one calls it;
When you come to share with your
brothers,
Your portion may be a storeroom.
If your god lets you have children,
They'll say: "We are in our father's
house."
Be a man hungry or sated in his
house,
It is his walls that enclose him.
Do not be a mindless person,
then your god will give you wealth.

-Ancient Egyptian Sage Ani

The culture of greed is antithetical to the age old wisdom of ethical wealth espoused by the Ancient Egyptian sages. Sage Amenemope speaks (above) of the fallacy that wealth is to be equated with happiness, stressing that peace of mind and closeness to the Divine are greater than physical wealth. Sage Ani reminds us (above) that too much reliance on the wealth of others (taking loans) allows others to control one's possessions and one's life. The culture of greed has as its foundation the idea that greed is a proper and useful motivational impetus to cause people to be industrious and productive as they seek to increase their individual wealth. The problem is that this philosophy cannot work to produce a balanced culture since there will always be some having more than others which necessarily must mean at the expense of others; such a condition necessarily leads to strife, for deep down all human beings know that it is fundamentally wrong to deprive others of their needs because we are essentially all connected in soul and spirit and thus when we deprive others we are depriving ourselves and leading ourselves to conscious or unconscious anguish and that creates negative *ariu* (karma) that will produce negative consequences in this or a future lifetime. Sharing is not only the correct manner in which human beings should live but it is also the only practical manner in which to coexist in harmony. Those who are wealthy (in physical terms) and who revel in their positions while allowing to be kept or actively keeping others in a state of material despair or low living standards, as well as those who worship the wealthy, thinking and hoping that they too may one day join their ranks, are sustaining the delusion of wealth as a harbinger of prosperity and happiness and are also sustaining the means of their own vexation (dissatisfaction, stress, anguish and misdirection in life) and preventing greater prosperity and spiritual fulfillment for themselves and others.

If people of means have a good name, and their face is benign, people will praise them even without their knowledge. Those whose hearts obey their bellies, however, ask for contempt instead of love. Their hearts are naked. Their bodies are unanointed. The great hearted are a gift from God. Those who are ruled by their appetites belong to the enemy."

-Ancient Egyptian Sage Ptahotep

(105) Do not refuse your oil jar to a stranger, Double it before your brothers.
(106) God prefers the person who honors the poor, to the one who worships the wealthy.

The love of God is better than the reverence of the nobleman.

-Ancient Egyptian Sage Amenemope

The aforesaid is specific advice on the treatment of family and strangers along with the proper attitude one should have towards those who are wealthier as well as the general advice for fostering a balanced society and stable economic condition. Now, since we are in a time of economic downfall the prudent path especially now, particularly for those who are in the financial markets or who are investors, is to "go to cash" or engage in short-term investing/trading. This is not a time to hold long-term investments but rather a time for short-term investments and or move to the necessity aspect of the economy (investing in areas where there will always be a need regardless of how bad things get). This means divesting from assets and debts so that when the full economic crisis ensues the wealth would not suffer the possible fate awaiting the economy that has been mishandled, that has suffered corruption and malfeasance. So, for example, those people who saw the signs of the economic downturn and sold their house and started renting in early 2007 missed the real estate crash due to the bursting of the real estate bubble (created by congress and the president relaxing or doing away with regulation of the rich and the Federal Reserve adding money to the economy that fueled speculation by Wall Street investors); they went to cash and preserved the physical wealth thereby. Those who sold their stock investments in July 2008 missed the crash in September and preserved their physical wealth thereby. Using the Great

Depression and all other market crashes including 2008 as examples, the value of assets falls dramatically until the economy finds a bottom and then rebuilds (if it has the capacity). This is due to an economic model that promotes booms and busts and allows speculative bubbles that distort the markets which then need to correct themselves by crashing periodically. If the market is not allowed to right itself normally and government leaders allow unrighteous printing of money and speculative bubbles by giving bailouts, or subsidies to certain industries, then the economy inflates without underlying value (stock market goes up while unemployment and the value of the dollar go down) and the economy may hobble along in a condition of malaise. Under such conditions the rich do not suffer but the other members of society do in the proportion to their wealth capacity. The unrighteous handling of the economy has occurred because of gutting the manufacturing base, hollowing out the middle class, allowing corporations to keep wages down while outsourcing jobs to countries with lower wages, printing money without real backing, creating inflation to suck the wealth out of the middle class and the poor, allowing bankers and the plutocracy to acquire that wealth, undermine the economy with unrighteous mortgages and exotic financial instruments sold around the world (multi-trillion dollar fraud), and allowing the wealthy people to hoard the wealth. These deeds and others have caused a situation in which while the stock markets may seem to rise, the economy will falter as more people are foreclosed, become unemployed and businesses cannot operate due to lack of funds (business loans) and lack of customers (due to the impoverished middle class and the poor). Nevertheless, the current condition of the economic imbalances is unprecedented and none of the economics experts can fully predict how negatively the economy will react and how it might recover or how long that might take.

This means that at some point, the economy will see more recession and will likely slip into a inflationary depression in which prices may go up due to the excessive money printing, as began to happen in the year 2008 with gasoline at $5 per gallon and food riots around the world, but the value of money will fall and many people will have less to spend due to having less employment and the higher cost of things. Therefore, the prudent thing to do in this case would be to maintain wealth is liquid forms while short term investing wealth in commodities or enterprises of necessity (like food industry, utilities, etc.) and or accumulate wealth and keeping it ready to be deployed when needed, just as was done in Ancient Egypt; when the Nile flood would be low in a year causing reduced harvests, the authorities would authorize the release of grain that was stored from the previous years that had normal or above average harvests, in order to prevent famine in the current year.

For those in business, especially those in enterprises that rely on customers that need jobs and a stable economy in order to have money to spend, the prudent thing to do would be to not take on long-term commitments that are unsecured, without proper collateral; not committing to expenses that may be fixed, like adding new equipment or building facilities that will depend on a stable or growing economy to be sustained. Right now the long-term outlook for the USA economy looks bleak in the sense that it will not have the growth it had in the previous 30 years which was due to bubbles created by malfeasance and were not real. The condition of the population is also bleak because no change has been made in the agenda of leaders (republicans and democrats) bent on impoverishing the middle class and the poor by empowering corporations, breaking up worker unions and convincing everyone that regulations on business produces less jobs (notice the constant and debilitating reliance on jobs from other people that allow the masses to be controlled and impoverished at will) and passing laws that shift the burden of taxes and healthcare to the middle class and the poor and away from the rich. The failed concept of Reaganomics tax cuts for the rich and less regulations for businesses, was not applied prior to 1980 and yet economically, the country prospered, while since 1980 the value of the dollar, and falling wages and benefits have been the mainstays of the economy while the rich get richer, in an evermore distorted and unbalance manner in reference to the rest of the population.

The Tech Bubble (1997-2000) and the housing bubble (2001-2007) were the last two artificial economic bubbles (false appreciation in asset values based on speculation) but the US Dollar and the National debt of the USA are also new bubbles that cannot be sustained. They cannot be sustained due to the loss of a manufacturing base, the hollowing out of the middle class, and trade policies that allow corporations to not pay fair wages and pay little or no taxes while taking the moneys from bailouts given by the government and investing them in emerging markets like China instead of making loans to small businesses and investing in the USA infrastructure with living wages so that ordinary people may be able to live a decent life and thereby contribute to the economic activity instead of becoming poor and contributing to the stagnation of the economy. All of this has led to a state of virtual bankruptcy of the USA and were it not for the status of world reserve currency the USA economy would have collapsed years ago. In the year 2008 China began to form an alternative world currency block, along with other Asian nations, to move away from the US Dollar and as that plan moves forward the US Dollar will lose its reserve status more and more and if the same malfeasance continues, the USA government's capacity to run huge deficits and sell treasury bonds to the world will go away, causing a full collapse of the economy; This all points to a stagnant USA economy for many years to come and the strong possibility of an economic downfall since the wealth of the majority has been taken out of the economy. So the rich will be alright but the middle class and poor will be destitute and languishing in a stagnant economy.

In contrast, if there were a full collapse of the economy the capacity of the USA government to perpetrate wars and sustain armed forces around the world to maintain an economic empire of world control would be reduced. Also, if corporate favoring bailouts and trade policies were reversed, the fraudulent debt on the middle class and the poor could be wiped clean and if the unfair wealth distribution imposed by the plutocrats through corporations, congress, presidents and judges were reversed, there could be a chance that the economy would turn around but that would take time to occur. In the mean time there is a possibility of social and political instability that might cause dangerous living conditions especially for those of modest means. Of course, there will always be some industries that will continue, like the food industry, the medical industry, etc. but most will be depressed and sustained by those with means, the upper middle class and the rich; yet, the living standards (quality of life) for the majority will be low and crime will be high.

Furthermore, those who are of like understanding should join in cooperative efforts to plan for such eventualities as a group. This will augment the individual efforts described above. Those who have the capacity to leave the country should plan for that eventuality as a stopgap, emergency measure and possible long-term strategy until the situation stabilizes. When that occurs (may take several years) then it may be prudent again to return and invest.

In the mean time, people may continue working and doing business if possible, until such eventualities as outlined above, may occur and resolve themselves. Those who still have assets that can be sold for a descent price may consider going to cash until the crisis passes. Another area to keep in mind is the investment of education. Those wishing to procreate may consider waiting until the situation stabilizes. For those who have children, they should encourage them to be educated in areas not susceptible to industries dependent upon discretionary income for obvious reasons; if customers are struggling they will spend first on necessities before extraneous desires. So education and careers should be pursued in areas of economic necessity. In reference to starting a business or investing in one, this may be prudent if the business is in a necessity industry.

Finally, there is a very high probability that the economy of the USA will slip further into deep recession and depression especially since the government gridlock between Democrats and Republicans (given the elections of 2010 increasing the power of right wing republicans) will either increase the Reaganomics policies (less regulation of business, more outsourcing, less manufacturing base, lower wages, breaking up unions, etc. to impoverish the masses and enrich the plutocrats) or prevent them (the politicians) from arriving at proper solutions (fiscal ethics, sound monetary policy, fair labor laws and trade policies) or even a temporary one, stimulus spending, all of which will leave, since the congress and president are in a state of gridlock, the Federal Reserve to lower interest rates and print money that will inflate the dollar without providing any investment (infrastructure and or manufacturing base) that would add value to the economy (thus diminishing the value of current wealth in dollar terms). The FED has already engaged in this process and the funds that were given to the banks, supposedly to allow them to lend to the domestic economy, have not been and will not be used by bankers to bolster the economy and meet the needs of small businesses and the majority population but rather to sure up their enterprises and bank accounts while investing in emerging (foreign) markets. Thus, eventually they and other foreigners will follow the plan of buying assets on the cheap when they see that the economy has found a bottom (as occurred in March 2009) which will restart the next cycle of boom (for financial markets-not for the general economy) until the next bust...

This downfall of assets will also temporarily affect all assets including gold and oil – commodities that are necessities. But when the immediate crisis passes there will be an opportunity to repurchase these again, at lower prices, for wealth preservation purposes and for medium to long-term investment purposes.

The Wisdom of Gold, Silver and Electrum Part 1

Q uestion:
Dear Sebai MAA, I have been watching the news and the price of gold recently went really high and the dollar seems to be falling a lot as you have been saying. The problem is that now gold is so expensive and I do not have funds to buy gold, or some of the other suggestions... and bills are tight. What can be done?

A Peace and blessings

nswer

The riddle of money can certainly be a challenging and perplexing issue especially in view of the great malfeasance that has led the society to the brink of economic disaster. The price of gold has increased much but it may rise much higher from where it is now before it is all over. Silver has been referred to as the "poor man's gold" because it is cheaper and the gains can be the same or more than gold (in relative monetary terms). Also silver can be used more easily as regular currency. So if you only have say a spare $40 per month you can get 2 silver coins. But even one at a time will develop into a golden movement towards wealth building.

Eventually you can build up a substantial fund. If the economy becomes more negative and or if the dollar continues to depreciate -as is expected, the value of the coins will increase substantially (but even if it does not appreciate it will hold on to the buying power or the value (at the time of the purchase) of the paper money it was bought with). At some point you will sell them and put the greater funds in a more advanced investment account. Other proper investments can be engaged with the ideal of the philosophy of wealth expressed in the wisdom of gold and silver, which may include, at this time, energy, commodities, etc. because when the economy falters and the currency falls, the real necessities increase in value. Do not neglect to consider cooperating with others of like mind to pool resources and employ assets in endeavors that may build wealth more quickly as a group than what might be possible individually. Nevertheless, either as an individual or as a group the ideal is the same.

On next page:

Figure 15: Akhenaten in his electrum chariot

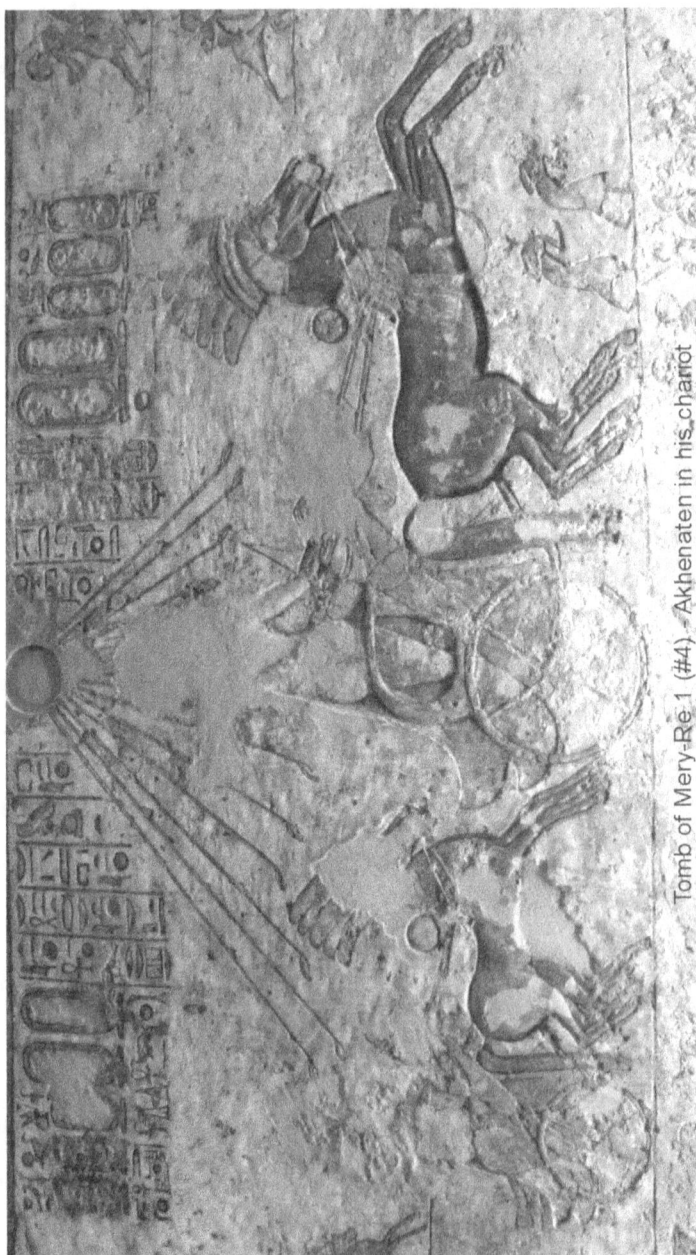

Tomb of Mery-Rē 1 (#4). - Akhenaten in his chariot

So you should take care of necessities first and then with whatever is left, the important thing right now is to save save save as much of your wealth as possible. Consider that if you were to put money away now in precious metals and foreign currencies and if the price of these increases (versus the US Dollar) you would be more easily able to pay off bills. So a prudent plan could be to pay minimums on your long-term debts and put the moneys you would use to pay extra on bills into gold, silver etc. and then wait until the depreciation of dollars occurs and then pay them off more easily, with assets and currencies of higher value and have wealth left over. So anything you can save will be to your benefit. Use coins or other programs as we have suggested, as outlined in the books *Collapse of Civilization and Death of American Empire* (2006) and *Dollar Crisis* (2008) and now the eBOOK *Malfeasance & Immorality* (2010) that are in keeping with Ancient Egyptian Economics contained in this volume. You should act now, doing whatever you can, before the prices go up more - think about it - every time the prices of gold and silver go up it means that the dollar is worth less and actually buys less - that is a sign of nominal inflation and what will come next? If you save your wealth it will be available later. Those who do not act are losing their wealth-as we speak. How much good will it does to have $10000 in the future that buys only $1000 worth of necessities? (In the future $10000 might only buy what you could buy today with $1000). That is what could happen; it may be referred to as inflation but it's in reality devaluation of the currency and in other words, loss of buying power, in other words, loss of wealth. The prudent thing to do is to protect wealth and whether or not a worse case scenario occurs you are saving wealth and building it instead of, like most people, acting as if "there is no problem, or leaders will figure it out or things will just get worse and we will have to live with it...etc." It does not make sense to trust in those who have demonstrated their unrighteousness or incompetence and not do what is within one's power to protect oneself...this is not the Kemetic way.

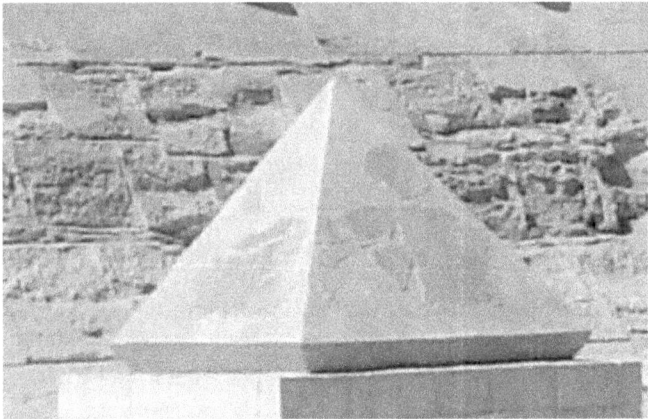

Figure 16: The restored pyramidon (Capstone) belonging to the Red Pyramid of Pharaoh Snoferu, at Dahshur, is now on permanent open air display beside the pyramid it was intended to surmount.

The Kemetic way is the way of gold, silver and electrum. Gold is the sun, the ever shining eternity that does not stop and is the source of life. Silver is the moon, the mind in which the sunlight reflects;

the moon fluctuates, has phases, movements and tasks. The sun is immovable, perennial and ever-present. Electrum is an alloy of gold and silver, the nexus between the two, the connection, nay, the union. Many people know of the use of gold and silver in Ancient Egypt but few know the mystery of electrum. Gold is the immortal part, the spirit, silver is for the mind and it's activities in the world of time and space and electrum is the bridge, that which allows our world to connect with that of the gods and goddesses. The Sage King Akhenaton rode in a chariot of electrum; a vehicle to take him to the glorious union. In the construction of the pyramids and obelisks the capstone (pyramidon),

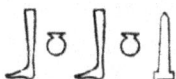

the ⌐σ⌐σ⌐ BenBen, the point between heaven and earth, the point where earth touches sky, was covered with what else? Electrum. We are to have pure mind, electrum, through practice of the disciplines of Maat philosophy and spiritual sensitivity through the practice of Egyptian Mysteries and meditation, to reflect the spirit, gold, in our mind, silver. So too in day to day life we should have pure currency (silver) to reflect the true power of wealth (gold) and not rely on the loans from others or the paper money of others.

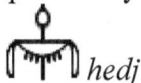

hedj

Figure 17: silver, was referred to as hedj

In the same way we should have pure currency to operate effectively in the world. Paper money is a shadow of real money; real money is silver and the power of silver is gold. Paper money has no real value unless it represents a storehouse of silver and gold. The combination of gold and silver is called "electrum".

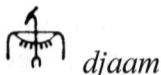 *djaam*

Figure 18: Electrum was called (djaam). It was a natural or artificial alloy composed of gold and silver. It came from Nubia, Punt, Emu and the mountains of the desert

We are to have purity of soul so as to operate effectively in Spirit. If we forget the gold in pursuit of the silver we may gain hollow wealth; wealth without aesthetic, without sensitivity, without compassion, a wealth of greed and dishonor, of fiendish nature. The wealth of gold is marked by glorious giving, concern for the well-being of all and judicious, scrupulous attention to the honor of gold which translates into the righteous and responsible usage of silver in day to day life.

 Nub

Figure 19: Nub (noob), the gold hieroglyph

Possessing gold is important in giving this "solar wealth" to the ever-changing events of life (silver). So, for this time and place we are concerned about the gold and silver and electrum in the study of the mysteries. In the world and in the management of fiscal and monetary affairs we are concerned with silver backed by gold. Therefore, one should allow the lucid soul (illuminated by spirit/gold) to manifest as wisdom and ethics in worldly endeavors, using silver currency, silver thoughtfulness, and silver intent to express purity as prudence, righteous action, intent and integrity in the world. In order to have silvery conscience that reflects golden spirit consciousness it is necessary to cultivate electrum, the *nexus* between silver and gold, earth and heaven, human/soul and spirit.

Figure 20: Gold, Silver and electrum and the Ancient Egyptian Obelisk

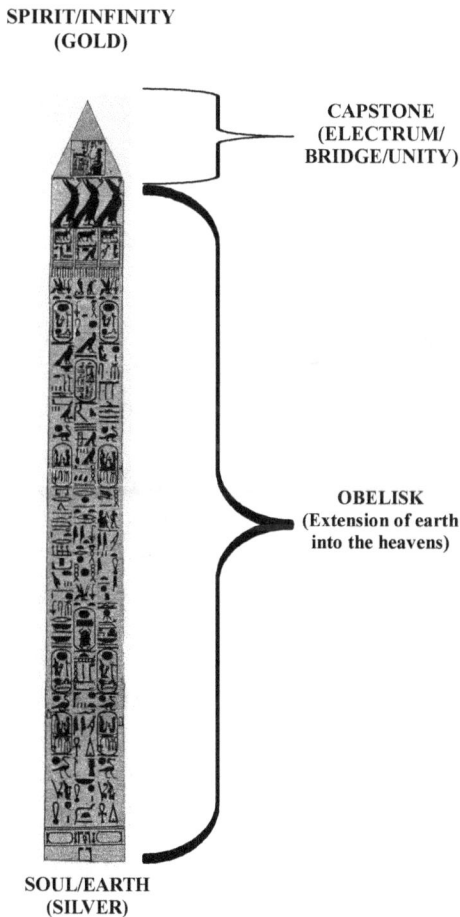

SPIRIT/INFINITY
(GOLD)

CAPSTONE
(ELECTRUM/
BRIDGE/UNITY)

OBELISK
(Extension of earth
into the heavens)

SOUL/EARTH
(SILVER)

The wisdom of gold, silver and electrum Part 2

Question: I have very modest means, how can I go about investing in gold and silver?

Answer:

Indeed, you may purchase 1 or 100 coins or more at a time according to your budget. If you cannot afford gold you can get silver. The prices will change daily and sometimes it goes up dramatically and sometimes down but over the longer term (years) the movement is pointing up because of the great malfeasance that has been perpetrated. But also because gold and silver have been regarded as money for the longest time and thus are considered safe harbors for wealth generally around the world. Yet throughout the fluctuations the storehouse of wealth remains. So the gold investment should be with a longer term view. The silver investment can be also seen with a long-term view but it can also be used in short-term ways like regular money.

The important thing is to get started and set an energetic tone that the Neteru (cosmic forces) of order and progress (Anpu, Maat, Sekhemit, Aset, etc.) will notice (resonate with) and favor (join with, augment) to your efforts to build wealth. This is a metaphysical mechanism of reciprocation but it is not as simple as doing a ritual or praying to the divine and then expecting something in return. In some circles this kind of teaching has been referred to as "The Secret" or by other names. However, "the secret" does not work for everyone. Getting what one wants in life is not just a matter of desiring it or even working for it; there is a teaching missing, which explains the cause of the failures. What those pundits do not explain is that a person cannot have what they desire if it is against their *ariu* until that *ariu* has been resolved. This is why "the secret" does not work for most people; they have worked for lifetimes in opposition to their present desires and therefore time is needed to resolve the effects of those past feelings, thoughts and actions as they are fructifying today; Hence the importance of ethical training in philosophy and mental/physical purification to understand the nature of the universe and of the inner self, beyond the personality, that is not susceptible to the personality's foibles and *ariu* (consequences of past actions). So there is no guarantee of the success of one's actions towards one's desires in the short term but over time they can be successful if there is perseverance and purity; however that time may span lifetimes. Additionally, even if there is success in achieving wealth there is no guarantee of retaining it unless there is true wealth of mind and soul. How many times have we seen people win lotteries only to squander the money away? Also, one's desires cannot be successful if they conflict with the *ariu* of others. For example, one person cannot inflict harm on another if that person's *ariu* is of a quality that is beyond allowing the person to get hurt. This points to the importance of purity so that the negative *ariu* either from one's own self or the desires of others or of the world may not control one's destiny or lead to negative outcomes. It is therefore important to work through subtle and gross *ariu* (actions, thoughts and feelings) through experiencing and working through varied worldly occurrences. In this way, the universe is set up such that all get the experiences, struggles and successes they need in order to grow and discover the nature of self without improper interference from others or the world.

Now, it is important to not only take a mental step but that needs to be followed up by a physical step if possible. If you desire to follow a path and you reflect and say that is good and I believe in that …this is the first and important step; then it is necessary to manifest that intent by taking steps in the direction of that desire. As the struggle progresses and as a person strives through setbacks, she/he gains experiences of failure and success and if they follow the teaching, their desire becomes more pure, more focused and more resonant. Then, if the desire is inline with the *ariu,* the thought/energy accumulated by the effort compels the desire to manifest, if it is not in contradiction with the *ariu* of others or of the world.

THE INSTRUCTION OF AMENEMOPE ON THE WISDOM OF WEALTH

(25)Do not set your heart on wealth,
There is no ignoring Fate and Destiny;
Do not let your heart go straying,
Every man comes to his hour.
Do not strain to seek increase,
(26)   What you have, let it suffice you.
If riches come to you by theft,
They will not stay the night with you.
Comes day they are not in your house,
Their place is seen but they are not there;
(27)Earth opened its mouth, leveled them, swallowed them,
And made them sink into dat.
They made a hole as big as their size,
And sank into the netherworld;
They made themselves wings like geese,
And flew away to the sky.

(28)Do not rejoice in wealth from theft,
Nor complain of being poor.
If the leading archer presses forward,
His company abandons him;

141

*(29)   The boat of the greedy is left (in) the
mud,
While the bark of the silent sails with the
wind.   Get into the habit of praying
sincerely to Aton (i.e. the solar Disk) as he
rises in the sky, saying,*

*Saying: "Grant me strength, well-being and
health";
He will give you your needs for this life,
And you will be safe from fear.*

So prosperity is not about desiring wealth for wealth
is a tool. The higher desire is to glorify the spirit in
the form of life. Wealth is necessary for the survival
and success of soul in the form of living beings. The
heart should not stray into wealth for wealth sake
(though one may become rich in the process), for
pleasure sake (though one may experience pleasure
along the path of life) or for fear of lack of wealth
(running for money so as to never experience want),
that boat eventually gets stuck in the mud
(dissatisfaction, unhappiness, darkening of the soul,
anxiety, dishonesty, etc.) of lower vibrating gross
worldly affairs that will never satisfy...no matter
how much money there may be. So one must take
care to not fall for the delusion of either the having
or the lacking of physical wealth. Physical gold and
silver are not the goal; they are the objective for
having sufficient resources to workout the mysteries

of life (the goal). So first realize that you yourself, the inner self, are the gold, the eternal spirit, and your life is the silver, the reflection of consciousness in time and space. As you unravel the mysteries of life and of spirit and harmonize your life and discover inner peace and successfully take care of the basic needs of life you are developing electrum, the connection between heaven and earth, that leads to spiritual enlightenment. Physical gold in the form of coins, nuggets, jewelry, etc, is coagulated sunlight, in essence, physical spirit. When the physical gold is used for negative deeds it is because the spirit gold inside the deeper recesses of the personality is clouded, submerged in the ocean of worldly desires and delusions. To the extent that the inner gold shines, to that extent the personality accomplishes golden deeds. Physical silver is coagulated thoughts that emanate from the radiance of gold. The silvery mind applies the wisdom of gold just as Lord Djehuty accomplishes the desires of Ra. This philosophy that speaks of such things is the electrum that enlightens about this wisdom. Electrum, which also manifests in the physical world as the alloy of gold and silver, is the mystic wisdom teaching, the practice of meditation and breath-work that allows a human being to connect the conscious mind to the transcendental recesses of the unconscious.

HTP
SMAA

143

Question: I am not familiar with investments, currencies, stocks, etc. How does one protect oneself from the economic crisis?

Answer:
You should find out all you can about the crisis and also consult books on the subject and if possible speak to people who know and work in this area. We do not give financial advice for specific investments but general advice that can set you on the path to understanding what needs to be done. You must decide on the course of action that is best for you as an individual. If you decide to join an investment club you can learn with others and research collectively the best strategies to safeguard your finances.

Firstly, you should not put all your funds in one place: diversification is a key to safety and survivability- Optimally, the best course is to keep moneys in different currencies, different countries and different forms (currency, precious metals, stocks, bonds of countries with sound finances, commodities, real goods.). The real estate you live in may be held in ownership status but due to current conditions, the better way to handle that asset might be to sell it and then rent and take the money and put it in safe places before the further real estate deflation occurs. Later, when conditions normalize, a purchase could be considered. Many people who can no longer sell are taking other action like taking out home equity loans and then taking the money and putting it away safely--the income they get from the investment they use to pay the mortgage and still have surplus because the investment pays higher interest than the mortgage. This action requires thought and research. There are a few forms of investment that are useful at this time: precious metals (gold and silver primarily), foreign currency, foreign stocks (in non-discretionary businesses-like utilities, medical, food, etc. -always attempting to invest in companies that are responsible to the environment and the community. It is easy to open a stock broker account to purchase foreign currency and stocks and electronic gold. Also, another method is -you can easily set up a foreign account to own gold and silver and have it stored offshore in a different country like Australia or England/Switzerland. It is prudent to keep a few coins hidden at home along with some cash-enough to last for 2 months of expenses (if there is no exchange for coins then it is not useful to keep them in hand -the forms mentioned above allow easy exchange for cash). It takes more effort but is also prudent (if there are substantial funds to save) to have the funds in completely foreign accounts in other countries so that there is no opportunity for it to be confiscated or otherwise disturbed by a corrupt banking system, chaotic government or breakdowns in the social order. The investments such as foreign stocks -that keep the money in foreign currency also produce income which will be worth more in terms of dollars -if the dollar collapses. Read the books for more details.[28]

---

[28] *Collapse of Civilization and Death of American Empire* (2006) and *Dollar Crisis* (2008) and now the eBOOK *Malfeasance & Immorality* (2010) www.Egyptianyoga.com/catalog

INDEX

Other Books From C M Books

P.O.Box 570459
Miami, Florida, 33257
(305) 378-6253 Fax: (305) 378-6253

This book is part of a series on the study and practice of Ancient Egyptian Yoga and Mystical Spirituality based on the writings of Dr. Muata Abhaya Ashby. They are also part of the Egyptian Yoga Course provided by the Sema Institute of Yoga. Below you will find a listing of the other books in this series. For more information send for the Egyptian Yoga Book-Audio-Video Catalog or the Egyptian Yoga Course Catalog.

Now you can study the teachings of Egyptian and Indian Yoga wisdom and Spirituality with the Egyptian Yoga Mystical Spirituality Series. The Egyptian Yoga Series takes you through the Initiation process and lead you to understand the mysteries of the soul and the Divine and to attain the highest goal of life: ENLIGHTENMENT. The *Egyptian Yoga Series*, takes you on an in depth study of Ancient Egyptian mythology and their inner mystical meaning. Each Book is prepared for the serious student of the mystical sciences and provides a study of the teachings along with exercises, assignments and projects to make the teachings understood and effective in real life. The Series is part of the Egyptian Yoga course but may be purchased even if you are not taking the course. The series is ideal for study groups.

Prices subject to change.

1. *EGYPTIAN YOGA: THE PHILOSOPHY OF ENLIGHTENMENT* An original, fully illustrated work, including hieroglyphs, detailing the meaning of the Egyptian mysteries, tantric yoga, psycho-spiritual and physical exercises. Egyptian Yoga is a guide to the practice of the highest spiritual philosophy which leads to absolute freedom from human misery and to

immortality. It is well known by scholars that Egyptian philosophy is the basis of Western and Middle Eastern religious philosophies such as *Christianity, Islam, Judaism,* the *Kabala,* and Greek philosophy, but what about Indian philosophy, Yoga and Taoism? What were the original teachings? How can they be practiced today? What is the source of pain and suffering in the world and what is the solution? Discover the deepest mysteries of the mind and universe within and outside of your self. 8.5" X 11" ISBN: 1-884564-01-1 Soft $19.95

2.   *EGYPTIAN YOGA: African Religion Volume 2-* Theban Theology U.S. In this long awaited sequel to *Egyptian Yoga: The Philosophy of Enlightenment* you will take a fascinating and enlightening journey back in time and discover the teachings which constituted the epitome of Ancient Egyptian spiritual wisdom. What are the disciplines which lead to the fulfillment of all desires? Delve into the three states of consciousness (waking, dream and deep sleep) and the fourth state which transcends them all, Neberdjer, "The Absolute." These teachings of the city of Waset (Thebes) were the crowning achievement of the Sages of Ancient Egypt. They establish the standard mystical keys for understanding the profound mystical symbolism of the Triad of human consciousness. ISBN 1-884564-39-9 $23.95

3.   *THE KEMETIC DIET: GUIDE TO HEALTH, DIET AND FASTING* Health issues have always been important to human beings since the beginning of time. The earliest records of history show that the art of healing was held in high esteem since the time of Ancient Egypt. In the early 20th century, medical doctors had almost attained the status of sainthood by the promotion of the idea that they alone were "scientists" while other healing modalities and traditional healers who did not follow the "scientific

method' were nothing but superstitious, ignorant charlatans who at best would take the money of their clients and at worst kill them with the unscientific "snake oils" and "irrational theories". In the late 20th century, the failure of the modern medical establishment's ability to lead the general public to good health, promoted the move by many in society towards "alternative medicine". Alternative medicine disciplines are those healing modalities which do not adhere to the philosophy of allopathic medicine. Allopathic medicine is what medical doctors practice by an large. It is the theory that disease is caused by agencies outside the body such as bacteria, viruses or physical means which affect the body. These can therefore be treated by medicines and therapies The natural healing method began in the absence of extensive technologies with the idea that all the answers for health may be found in nature or rather, the deviation from nature. Therefore, the health of the body can be restored by correcting the aberration and thereby restoring balance. This is the area that will be covered in this volume. Allopathic techniques have their place in the art of healing. However, we should not forget that the body is a grand achievement of the spirit and built into it is the capacity to maintain itself and heal itself. Ashby, Muata ISBN: 1-884564-49-6 $28.95

4.   INITIATION INTO EGYPTIAN YOGA Shedy: Spiritual discipline or program, to go deeply into the mysteries, to study the mystery teachings and literature profoundly, to penetrate the mysteries. You will learn about the mysteries of initiation into the teachings and practice of Yoga and how to become an Initiate of the mystical sciences. This insightful manual is the first in a series which introduces you to the goals of daily spiritual and yoga practices: Meditation, Diet, Words of Power and the ancient wisdom teachings. 8.5" X 11" ISBN 1-884564-02-X Soft Cover $24.95 U.S.

5. *THE AFRICAN ORIGINS OF CIVILIZATION,
    RELIGION AND YOGA SPIRITUALITY AND
    ETHICS PHILOSOPHY* HARD COVER EDITION
    Part 1, Part 2, Part 3 in one volume 683 Pages Hard
    Cover First Edition Three volumes in one. Over the
    past several years I have been asked to put together in
    one volume the most important evidences showing
    the correlations and common teachings between
    Kamitan (Ancient Egyptian) culture and religion and
    that of India. The questions of the history of Ancient
    Egypt, and the latest archeological evidences
    showing civilization and culture in Ancient Egypt
    and its spread to other countries, has intrigued many
    scholars as well as mystics over the years. Also, the
    possibility that Ancient Egyptian Priests and
    Priestesses migrated to Greece, India and other
    countries to carry on the traditions of the Ancient
    Egyptian Mysteries, has been speculated over the
    years as well. In chapter 1 of the book *Egyptian Yoga
    The Philosophy of Enlightenment,* 1995, I first
    introduced the deepest comparison between Ancient
    Egypt and India that had been brought forth up to that
    time. Now, in the year 2001 this new book, *THE
    AFRICAN ORIGINS OF CIVILIZATION, MYSTICAL
    RELIGION AND YOGA PHILOSOPHY,* more fully
    explores the motifs, symbols and philosophical
    correlations between Ancient Egyptian and Indian
    mysticism and clearly shows not only that Ancient
    Egypt and India were connected culturally but also
    spiritually. How does this knowledge help the
    spiritual aspirant? This discovery has great
    importance for the Yogis and mystics who follow the
    philosophy of Ancient Egypt and the mysticism of
    India. It means that India has a longer history and
    heritage than was previously understood. It shows
    that the mysteries of Ancient Egypt were essentially a
    yoga tradition which did not die but rather developed
    into the modern day systems of Yoga technology of
    India. It further shows that African culture developed

Yoga Mysticism earlier than any other civilization in history. All of this expands our understanding of the unity of culture and the deep legacy of Yoga, which stretches into the distant past, beyond the Indus Valley civilization, the earliest known high culture in India as well as the Vedic tradition of Aryan culture. Therefore, Yoga culture and mysticism is the oldest known tradition of spiritual development and Indian mysticism is an extension of the Ancient Egyptian mysticism. By understanding the legacy which Ancient Egypt gave to India the mysticism of India is better understood and by comprehending the heritage of Indian Yoga, which is rooted in Ancient Egypt the Mysticism of Ancient Egypt is also better understood. This expanded understanding allows us to prove the underlying kinship of humanity, through the common symbols, motifs and philosophies which are not disparate and confusing teachings but in reality expressions of the same study of truth through metaphysics and mystical realization of Self. (HARD COVER) ISBN: 1-884564-50-X $45.00 U.S.   81/2" X 11"

6.   *AFRICAN ORIGINS BOOK 1 PART 1* African Origins of African Civilization, Religion, Yoga Mysticism and Ethics Philosophy-Soft Cover $24.95 ISBN: 1-884564-55-0

7.   *AFRICAN ORIGINS BOOK 2 PART 2* African Origins of Western Civilization, Religion and Philosophy (Soft) -Soft Cover $24.95 ISBN: 1-884564-56-9

8.   *EGYPT AND INDIA* AFRICAN ORIGINS OF *Eastern Civilization, Religion, Yoga Mysticism and Philosophy*-Soft Cover $29.95 (Soft) ISBN: 1-884564-57-7

9.   *THE MYSTERIES OF ISIS: The Ancient Egyptian Philosophy of Self-Realization* - There are several paths to discover the Divine and the mysteries of the higher Self. This volume details the mystery teachings of the goddess Aset (Isis) from Ancient Egypt- the path of wisdom. It includes the teachings of her temple and the disciplines that are enjoined for the initiates of the temple of Aset as they were given in ancient times. Also, this book includes the teachings of the main myths of Aset that lead a human being to spiritual enlightenment and immortality. Through the study of ancient myth and the illumination of initiatic understanding the idea of God is expanded from the mythological comprehension to the metaphysical. Then this metaphysical understanding is related to you, the student, so as to begin understanding your true divine nature. ISBN 1-884564-24-0 $22.99

10.   *EGYPTIAN PROVERBS:*   collection of —Ancient Egyptian Proverbs and Wisdom Teachings -How to live according to MAAT Philosophy. Beginning Meditation. All proverbs are indexed for easy searches. For the first time in one volume, —— Ancient Egyptian Proverbs, wisdom teachings and meditations, fully illustrated with hieroglyphic text and symbols. EGYPTIAN PROVERBS is a unique collection of knowledge and wisdom which you can put into practice today and transform your life. $14.95 U.S   ISBN: 1-884564-00-3

11.   *GOD OF LOVE: THE PATH OF DIVINE LOVE The Process of Mystical Transformation and The Path of Divine Love*   This Volume focuses on the ancient wisdom teachings of "Neter Merri" –the Ancient Egyptian philosophy of Divine Love and how to use them in a scientific process for self-transformation. Love is one of the most powerful human emotions. It is also the source of Divine feeling that unifies God

and the individual human being. When love is fragmented and diminished by egoism the Divine connection is lost. The Ancient tradition of Neter Merri leads human beings back to their Divine connection, allowing them to discover their innate glorious self that is actually Divine and immortal. This volume will detail the process of transformation from ordinary consciousness to cosmic consciousness through the integrated practice of the teachings and the path of Devotional Love toward the Divine. 5.5"x 8.5" ISBN 1-884564-11-9 $22.95

12. *INTRODUCTION TO MAAT PHILOSOPHY: Spiritual Enlightenment Through the Path of Virtue* Known commonly as Karma in India, the teachings of MAAT contain an extensive philosophy based on ariu (deeds) and their fructification in the form of shai and renenet (fortune and destiny, leading to Meskhenet (fate in a future birth) for living virtuously and with orderly wisdom are explained and the student is to begin practicing the precepts of Maat in daily life so as to promote the process of purification of the heart in preparation for the judgment of the soul. This judgment will be understood not as an event that will occur at the time of death but as an event that occurs continuously, at every moment in the life of the individual. The student will learn how to become allied with the forces of the Higher Self and to thereby begin cleansing the mind (heart) of impurities so as to attain a higher vision of reality. ISBN 1-884564-20-8 $22.99

13. *MEDITATION The Ancient Egyptian Path to Enlightenment* Many people do not know about the rich history of meditation practice in Ancient Egypt. This volume outlines the theory of meditation and presents the Ancient Egyptian Hieroglyphic text which give instruction as to the nature of the mind

and its three modes of expression. It also presents the texts which give instruction on the practice of meditation for spiritual Enlightenment and unity with the Divine. This volume allows the reader to begin practicing meditation by explaining, in easy to understand terms, the simplest form of meditation and working up to the most advanced form which was practiced in ancient times and which is still practiced by yogis around the world in modern times. ISBN 1-884564-27-7 $22.99

14. *THE GLORIOUS LIGHT MEDITATION* TECHNIQUE OF ANCIENT EGYPT New for the year 2000. This volume is based on the earliest known instruction in history given for the practice of formal meditation. Discovered by Dr. Muata Ashby, it is inscribed on the walls of the Tomb of Seti I in Thebes Egypt. This volume details the philosophy and practice of this unique system of meditation originated in Ancient Egypt and the earliest practice of meditation known in the world which occurred in the most advanced African Culture. ISBN: 1-884564-15-1 $16.95 (PB)

15. *THE SERPENT POWER: The Ancient Egyptian Mystical Wisdom of the Inner Life Force.* This Volume specifically deals with the latent life Force energy of the universe and in the human body, its control and sublimation. How to develop the Life Force energy of the subtle body. This Volume will introduce the esoteric wisdom of the science of how virtuous living acts in a subtle and mysterious way to cleanse the latent psychic energy conduits and vortices of the spiritual body. ISBN 1-884564-19-4 $22.95

16. *EGYPTIAN YOGA The Postures of The Gods and Goddesses* Discover the physical postures and exercises practiced thousands of years ago in Ancient Egypt which are today known as Yoga exercises.

Discover the history of the postures and how they were transferred from Ancient Egypt in Africa to India through Buddhist Tantrism. Then practice the postures as you discover the mythic teaching that originally gave birth to the postures and was practiced by the Ancient Egyptian priests and priestesses. This work is based on the pictures and teachings from the Creation story of Ra, The Asarian Resurrection Myth and the carvings and reliefs from various Temples in Ancient Egypt 8.5" X 11" ISBN 1-884564-10-0 Soft Cover $21.95 Exercise video $20

17. *SACRED SEXUALITY: EGYPTIAN TANTRA YOGA: The Art of Sex* Sublimation and Universal Consciousness This Volume will expand on the male and female principles within the human body and in the universe and further detail the sublimation of sexual energy into spiritual energy. The student will study the deities Min and Hathor, Asar and Aset, Geb and Nut and discover the mystical implications for a practical spiritual discipline. This Volume will also focus on the Tantric aspects of Ancient Egyptian and Indian mysticism, the purpose of sex and the mystical teachings of sexual sublimation which lead to self-knowledge and Enlightenment. 5.5"x 8.5" ISBN 1-884564-03-8 $24.95

18. *AFRICAN RELIGION Volume 4: ASARIAN THEOLOGY: RESURRECTING OSIRIS* The path of Mystical Awakening and the Keys to Immortality NEW REVISED AND EXPANDED EDITION! The Ancient Sages created stories based on human and superhuman beings whose struggles, aspirations, needs and desires ultimately lead them to discover their true Self. The myth of Aset, Asar and Heru is no exception in this area. While there is no one source where the entire story may be found, pieces of it are inscribed in various ancient Temples walls, tombs,

steles and papyri. For the first time available, the complete myth of Asar, Aset and Heru has been compiled from original Ancient Egyptian, Greek and Coptic Texts. This epic myth has been richly illustrated with reliefs from the Temple of Heru at Edfu, the Temple of Aset at Philae, the Temple of Asar at Abydos, the Temple of Hathor at Denderah and various papyri, inscriptions and reliefs. Discover the myth which inspired the teachings of the *Shetaut Neter* (Egyptian Mystery System - Egyptian Yoga) and the Egyptian Book of Coming Forth By Day. Also, discover the three levels of Ancient Egyptian Religion, how to understand the mysteries of the Duat or Astral World and how to discover the abode of the Supreme in the Amenta, *The Other World* The ancient religion of Asar, Aset and Heru, if properly understood, contains all of the elements necessary to lead the sincere aspirant to attain immortality through inner self-discovery. This volume presents the entire myth and explores the main mystical themes and rituals associated with the myth for understating human existence, creation and the way to achieve spiritual emancipation - *Resurrection.* The Asarian myth is so powerful that it influenced and is still having an effect on the major world religions. Discover the origins and mystical meaning of the Christian Trinity, the Eucharist ritual and the ancient origin of the birthday of Jesus Christ. Soft Cover ISBN: 1-884564-27-5 $24.95

19.   *THE EGYPTIAN BOOK OF THE DEAD MYSTICISM OF THE PERT EM HERU* " I Know myself, I know myself, I am One With God!–From the Pert Em Heru "The Ru Pert em Heru" or "Ancient Egyptian Book of The Dead," or "Book of Coming Forth By Day" as it is more popularly known, has fascinated the world since the successful translation of Ancient Egyptian hieroglyphic scripture over 150 years ago. The astonishing writings in it reveal that the Ancient Egyptians

believed in life after death and in an ultimate destiny to discover the Divine. The elegance and aesthetic beauty of the hieroglyphic text itself has inspired many see it as an art form in and of itself. But is there more to it than that? Did the Ancient Egyptian wisdom contain more than just aphorisms and hopes of eternal life beyond death? In this volume Dr. Muata Ashby, the author of over 25 books on Ancient Egyptian Yoga Philosophy has produced a new translation of the original texts which uncovers a mystical teaching underlying the sayings and rituals instituted by the Ancient Egyptian Sages and Saints. "Once the philosophy of Ancient Egypt is understood as a mystical tradition instead of as a religion or primitive mythology, it reveals its secrets which if practiced today will lead anyone to discover the glory of spiritual self-discovery. The Pert em Heru is in every way comparable to the Indian Upanishads or the Tibetan Book of the Dead." □ $28.95   ISBN# 1-884564-28-3 Size: 8½" X 11

20.   *African Religion VOL. 1- ANUNIAN THEOLOGY THE MYSTERIES OF RA* The Philosophy of Anu and The Mystical Teachings of The Ancient Egyptian Creation Myth Discover the mystical teachings contained in the Creation Myth and the gods and goddesses who brought creation and human beings into existence. The Creation myth of Anu is the source of Anunian Theology but also of the other main theological systems of Ancient Egypt that also influenced other world religions including Christianity, Hinduism and Buddhism. The Creation Myth holds the key to understanding the universe and for attaining spiritual Enlightenment. ISBN: 1-884564-38-0 $19.95

21.   *African Religion VOL 3: Memphite Theology: MYSTERIES OF MIND* Mystical Psychology & Mental Health for Enlightenment and Immortality

based on the Ancient Egyptian Philosophy of Menefer -Mysticism of Ptah, Egyptian Physics and Yoga Metaphysics and the Hidden properties of Matter. This volume uncovers the mystical psychology of the Ancient Egyptian wisdom teachings centering on the philosophy of the Ancient Egyptian city of Menefer (Memphite Theology). How to understand the mind and how to control the senses and lead the mind to health, clarity and mystical self-discovery. This Volume will also go deeper into the philosophy of God as creation and will explore the concepts of modern science and how they correlate with ancient teachings. This Volume will lay the ground work for the understanding of the philosophy of universal consciousness and the initiatic/yogic insight into who or what is God? ISBN 1-884564-07-0 $22.95

22. *AFRICAN RELIGION VOLUME 5: THE GODDESS AND THE EGYPTIAN MYSTERIESTHE PATH OF THE GODDESS THE GODDESS PATH* The Secret Forms of the Goddess and the Rituals of Resurrection The Supreme Being may be worshipped as father or as mother. *Ushet Rekhat* or *Mother Worship,* is the spiritual process of worshipping the Divine in the form of the Divine Goddess. It celebrates the most important forms of the Goddess including *Nathor, Maat, Aset, Arat, Amentet and Hathor* and explores their mystical meaning as well as the rising of *Sirius,* the star of Aset (Aset) and the new birth of Hor (Heru). The end of the year is a time of reckoning, reflection and engendering a new or renewed positive movement toward attaining spiritual Enlightenment. The Mother Worship devotional meditation ritual, performed on five days during the month of December and on New Year's Eve, is based on the Ushet Rekhit. During the ceremony, the cosmic forces, symbolized by Sirius - and the constellation of Orion ---, are harnessed through the understanding and devotional attitude of the participant. This

propitiation draws the light of wisdom and health to all those who share in the ritual, leading to prosperity and wisdom. $14.95 ISBN 1-884564-18-6

23. *THE MYSTICAL JOURNEY FROM JESUS TO CHRIST* Discover the ancient Egyptian origins of Christianity before the Catholic Church and learn the mystical teachings given by Jesus to assist all humanity in becoming Christlike. Discover the secret meaning of the Gospels that were discovered in Egypt. Also discover how and why so many Christian churches came into being. Discover that the Bible still holds the keys to mystical realization even though its original writings were changed by the church. Discover how to practice the original teachings of Christianity which leads to the Kingdom of Heaven. $24.95   ISBN# 1-884564-05-4 size: 8½" X 11"

24. *THE STORY OF ASAR, ASET AND HERU:* An Ancient Egyptian Legend (For Children)   Now for the first time, the most ancient myth of Ancient Egypt comes alive for children. Inspired by the books *The Asarian Resurrection: The Ancient Egyptian Bible* and *The Mystical Teachings of The Asarian Resurrection, The Story of Asar, Aset and Heru* is an easy to understand and thrilling tale which inspired the children of Ancient Egypt to aspire to greatness and righteousness.   If you and your child have enjoyed stories like *The Lion King* and *Star Wars you will love The Story of Asar, Aset and Heru.* Also, if you know the story of Jesus and Krishna you will discover than Ancient Egypt had a similar myth and that this myth carries important spiritual teachings for living a fruitful and fulfilling life. This book may be used along with *The Parents Guide To The Asarian Resurrection Myth: How to Teach Yourself and Your Child the Principles of Universal Mystical Religion.* The guide provides some background to the Asarian

Resurrection myth and it also gives insight into the mystical teachings contained in it which you may introduce to your child. It is designed for parents who wish to grow spiritually with their children and it serves as an introduction for those who would like to study the Asarian Resurrection Myth in depth and to practice its teachings. 8.5" X 11"   ISBN: 1-884564-31-3 $12.95

25.   *THE PARENTS GUIDE TO THE AUSARIAN RESURRECTION MYTH:*   How to Teach Yourself and Your Child the Principles of Universal Mystical Religion.   This insightful manual brings for the timeless wisdom of the ancient through the Ancient Egyptian myth of Asar, Aset and Heru and the mystical teachings contained in it for parents who want to guide their children to understand and practice the teachings of mystical spirituality. This manual may be used with the children's storybook *The Story of Asar, Aset and Heru* by Dr. Muata Abhaya Ashby.   ISBN: 1-884564-30-5 $16.95

26.   *HEALING THE CRIMINAL HEART.* Introduction to Maat Philosophy, Yoga and Spiritual Redemption Through the Path of Virtue   Who is a criminal? Is there such a thing as a criminal heart? What is the source of evil and sinfulness and is there any way to rise above it? Is there redemption for those who have committed sins, even the worst crimes?   Ancient Egyptian mystical psychology holds important answers to these questions. Over ten thousand years ago mystical psychologists, the Sages of Ancient Egypt, studied and charted the human mind and spirit and laid out a path which will lead to spiritual redemption, prosperity and Enlightenment.   This introductory volume brings forth the teachings of the Asarian Resurrection, the most important myth of Ancient Egypt, with relation to the faults of human existence: anger, hatred, greed, lust, animosity,

discontent, ignorance, egoism jealousy, bitterness, and a myriad of psycho-spiritual ailments which keep a human being in a state of negativity and adversity ISBN: 1-884564-17-8 $15.95

27.   *TEMPLE RITUAL OF THE ANCIENT EGYPTIAN MYSTERIES--THEATER & DRAMA OF THE ANCIENT EGYPTIAN MYSTERIES*: Details the practice of the mysteries and ritual program of the temple and the philosophy an practice of the ritual of the mysteries, its purpose and execution. Featuring the Ancient Egyptian stage play-"The Enlightenment of Hathor' Based on an Ancient Egyptian Drama, The original Theater -Mysticism of the Temple of Hetheru 1-884564-14-3 $19.95   By Dr. Muata Ashby

28.   *GUIDE TO PRINT ON DEMAND: SELF-PUBLISH FOR PROFIT,* SPIRITUAL FULFILLMENT AND SERVICE TO HUMANITY Everyone asks us how we produced so many books in such a short time. Here are the secrets to writing and producing books that uplift humanity and how to get them printed for a fraction of the regular cost. Anyone can become an author even if they have limited funds. All that is necessary is the willingness to learn how the printing and book business work and the desire to follow the special instructions given here for preparing your manuscript format. Then you take your work directly to the non-traditional companies who can produce your books for less than the traditional book printer can. ISBN: 1-884564-40-2 $16.95 U. S.

29.   *Egyptian Mysteries: Vol. 1,* Shetaut Neter What are the Mysteries? For thousands of years the spiritual tradition of Ancient Egypt, S*hetaut Neter,* "The Egyptian Mysteries," "The Secret Teachings," have fascinated, tantalized and amazed the world. At one time exalted and recognized as the highest culture of the world, by Africans, Europeans, Asiatics, Hindus,

Buddhists and other cultures of the ancient world, in time it was shunned by the emerging orthodox world religions. Its temples desecrated, its philosophy maligned, its tradition spurned, its philosophy dormant in the mystical *Medu Neter*, the mysterious hieroglyphic texts which hold the secret symbolic meaning that has scarcely been discerned up to now. What are the secrets of *Nehast* {spiritual awakening and emancipation, resurrection}. More than just a literal translation, this volume is for awakening to the secret code *Shetitu* of the teaching which was not deciphered by Egyptologists, nor could be understood by ordinary spiritualists. This book is a reinstatement of the original science made available for our times, to the reincarnated followers of Ancient Egyptian culture and the prospect of spiritual freedom to break the bonds of *Khemn,* "ignorance," and slavery to evil forces: *Såaa* . ISBN: 1-884564-41-0 $19.99

30.   *EGYPTIAN MYSTERIES VOL 2:* Dictionary of Gods and Goddesses This book is about the mystery of neteru, the gods and goddesses of Ancient Egypt (Kamit, Kemet). Neteru means "Gods and Goddesses." But the Neterian teaching of Neteru represents more than the usual limited modern day concept of "divinities" or "spirits." The Neteru of Kamit are also metaphors, cosmic principles and vehicles for the enlightening teachings of Shetaut Neter (Ancient Egyptian-African Religion). Actually they are the elements for one of the most advanced systems of spirituality ever conceived in human history. Understanding the concept of neteru provides a firm basis for spiritual evolution and the pathway for viable culture, peace on earth and a healthy human society.   Why is it important to have gods and goddesses in our lives? In order for spiritual evolution to be possible, once a human being has accepted that there is existence after death and there is a transcendental being who exists beyond time and

space knowledge, human beings need a connection to that which transcends the ordinary experience of human life in time and space and a means to understand the transcendental reality beyond the mundane reality. ISBN: 1-884564-23-2 $21.95

31.   *EGYPTIAN MYSTERIES VOL. 3* The Priests and Priestesses of Ancient Egypt This volume details the path of Neterian priesthood, the joys, challenges and rewards of advanced Neterian life, the teachings that allowed the priests and priestesses to manage the most long lived civilization in human history and how that path can be adopted today; for those who want to tread the path of the Clergy of Shetaut Neter. ISBN: 1-884564-53-4 $24.95

32.   *The War of Heru and Set:* The Struggle of Good and Evil for Control of the World and The Human Soul This volume contains a novelized version of the Asarian Resurrection myth that is based on the actual scriptures presented in the Book Asarian Religion (old name –Resurrecting Osiris). This volume is prepared in the form of a screenplay and can be easily adapted to be used as a stage play. Spiritual seeking is a mythic journey that has many emotional highs and lows, ecstasies and depressions, victories and frustrations. This is the War of Life that is played out in the myth as the struggle of Heru and Set and those are mythic characters that represent the human Higher and Lower self. How to understand the war and emerge victorious in the journey o life? The ultimate victory and fulfillment can be experienced, which is not changeable or lost in time. The purpose of myth is to convey the wisdom of life through the story of divinities who show the way to overcome the challenges and foibles of life. In this volume the feelings and emotions of the characters of the myth have been highlighted to show the deeply rich texture of the Ancient Egyptian myth. This myth contains deep spiritual teachings and insights into the nature

of self, of God and the mysteries of life and the means to discover the true meaning of life and thereby achieve the true purpose of life. To become victorious in the battle of life means to become the King (or Queen) of Egypt.Have you seen movies like The Lion King, Hamlet, The Odyssey, or The Little Buddha? These have been some of the most popular movies in modern times. The Sema Institute of Yoga is dedicated to researching and presenting the wisdom and culture of ancient Africa. The Script is designed to be produced as a motion picture but may be addapted for the theater as well. $21.95 copyright 1998 By Dr. Muata Ashby ISBN 1-8840564-44-5

33. *AFRICAN DIONYSUS: FROM EGYPT TO GREECE:* The Kamitan Origins of Greek Culture and Religion ISBN: 1-884564-47-X FROM EGYPT TO GREECE This insightful manual is a reference to Ancient Egyptian mythology and philosophy and its correlation to what later became known as Greek and Rome mythology and philosophy. It outlines the basic tenets of the mythologies and shoes the ancient origins of Greek culture in Ancient Egypt. This volume also documents the origins of the Greek alphabet in Egypt as well as Greek religion, myth and philosophy of the gods and goddesses from Egypt from the myth of Atlantis and archaic period with the Minoans to the Classical period. This volume also acts as a resource for Colleges students who would like to set up fraternities and sororities based on the original Ancient Egyptian principles of Sheti and Maat philosophy. ISBN: 1-884564-47-X $22.95 U.S.

34. *THE FORTY TWO PRECEPTS OF MAAT, THE PHILOSOPHY OF RIGHTEOUS ACTION AND THE ANCIENT EGYPTIAN WISDOM TEXTS* ADVANCED STUDIES This manual is designed for use with the 1998 Maat Philosophy Class conducted by Dr. Muata Ashby. This is a detailed study of Maat Philosophy. It contains a compilation of the 42 laws or precepts of

Maat and the corresponding principles which they represent along with the teachings of the ancient Egyptian Sages relating to each. Maat philosophy was the basis of Ancient Egyptian society and government as well as the heart of Ancient Egyptian myth and spirituality. Maat is at once a goddess, a cosmic force and a living social doctrine, which promotes social harmony and thereby paves the way for spiritual evolution in all levels of society. ISBN: 1-884564-48-8 $16.95 U.S.

35.   *THE SECRET LOTUS: Poetry of Enlightenment*
Discover the mystical sentiment of the Kemetic teaching as expressed through the poetry of Sebai Muata Ashby. The teaching of spiritual awakening is uniquely experienced when the poetic sensibility is present. This first volume contains the poems written between 1996 and 2003. **1-884564--16 -X $16.99**

36. The Ancient Egyptian Buddha: The Ancient Egyptian Origins of Buddhism
This book is a compilation of several sections of a larger work, a book by the name of African Origins of Civilization, Religion, Yoga Mysticism and Ethics Philosophy. It also contains some additional evidences not contained in the larger work that demonstrate the correlation between Ancient Egyptian Religion and Buddhism. This book is one of several compiled short volumes that has been compiled so as to facilitate access to specific subjects contained in the larger work which is over 680 pages long. These short and small volumes have been specifically designed to cover one subject in a brief and low cost format. This present volume, The Ancient Egyptian Buddha: The Ancient Egyptian Origins of Buddhism, formed one subject in the larger work; actually it was one chapter of the larger work. However, this volume has some new additional evidences and comparisons of Buddhist and Neterian (Ancient Egyptian) philosophies not previously discussed. It was felt that this subject needed to be discussed because even in the early 21st century, the idea persists that Buddhism originated only in India independently. Yet there is

ample evidence from ancient writings and perhaps more importantly, iconographical evidences from the Ancient Egyptians and early Buddhists themselves that prove otherwise. This handy volume has been designed to be accessible to young adults and all others who would like to have an easy reference with documentation on this important subject. This is an important subject because the frame of reference with which we look at a culture depends strongly on our conceptions about its origins. in this case, if we look at the Buddhism as an Asiatic religion we would treat it and it's culture in one way. If we id as African [Ancient Egyptian] we not only would see it in a different light but we also must ascribe Africa with a glorious legacy that matches any other culture in human history and gave rise to one of the present day most important religious philosophies. We would also look at the culture and philosophies of the Ancient Egyptians as having African insights that offer us greater depth into the Buddhist philosophies. Those insights inform our knowledge about other African traditions and we can also begin to understand in a deeper way the effect of Ancient Egyptian culture on African culture and also on the Asiatic as well. We would also be able to discover the glorious and wondrous teaching of mystical philosophy that Ancient Egyptian Shetaut Neter religion offers, that is as powerful as any other mystic system of spiritual philosophy in the world today. ISBN: 1-884564-61-5 $28.95

37. The Death of American Empire: Neo-conservatism, Theocracy, Economic Imperialism, Environmental Disaster and the Collapse of Civilization

This work is a collection of essays relating to social and economic, leadership, and ethics, ecological and religious issues that are facing the world today in order to understand the course of history that has led humanity to its present condition and then arrive at positive solutions that will lead to better outcomes for all humanity. It surveys the development and decline of major empires throughout history and focuses on the creation of American Empire along with the social, political and economic policies that led to the prominence of the United States of America as a Superpower including the rise of the political control of the neo-con political philosophy including militarism and the military industrial complex in American politics and the rise of the religious right into and American Theocracy movement. This volume details, through historical and current events, the psychology behind the dominance of western culture in world politics through the "Superpower Syndrome Mandatory Conflict Complex" that drives the Superpower culture to establish itself above all others and then act hubristically to dominate world culture through legitimate influences as well as coercion, media censorship and misinformation leading to international hegemony and world conflict. This volume also details the financial policies that gave rise to American prominence in the global economy, especially after World War II, and promoted American preeminence over the world economy through Globalization as well as the environmental policies, including the oil economy, that are promoting degradation of the world ecology and contribute to the decline of America as an Empire culture. This volume finally explores the factors pointing to the decline of the American Empire economy and imperial power and what to expect in the aftermath of American prominence and how to survive the decline while at the same time promoting policies and social-economic-religious-political changes that are needed in order to promote the emergence of a beneficial and sustainable culture. **$25.95soft** 1-884564-25-9, Hard Cover **$29.95soft** 1-884564-45-3

38. The African Origins of Hatha Yoga: And its Ancient Mystical Teaching

The subject of this present volume, The Ancient Egyptian Origins of Yoga Postures, formed one subject in the larger works, African Origins of Civilization Religion, Yoga Mysticism and Ethics Philosophy and the Book Egypt and India is the section of the book African Origins of Civilization. Those works contain the collection of all correlations between Ancient Egypt and India. This volume also contains some additional information not contained in the previous work. It was felt that this subject needed to be discussed more directly, being treated in one volume, as opposed to being contained in the larger work along with other subjects, because even in the early 21st century, the idea persists that the Yoga and specifically, Yoga Postures, were invented and developed only in India. The Ancient Egyptians were peoples originally from Africa who were, in ancient times, colonists in India. Therefore it is no surprise that many Indian traditions including religious and Yogic, would be found earlier in Ancient Egypt. Yet there is ample evidence from ancient writings and perhaps more importantly, iconographical evidences from the Ancient Egyptians themselves and the Indians themselves that prove the connection between Ancient Egypt and India as well as the existence of a discipline of Yoga Postures in Ancient Egypt long before its practice in India. This handy volume has been designed to be accessible to young adults and all others who would like to have an easy reference with documentation on this important subject. This is an important subject because the frame of reference with which we look at a culture depends strongly on our conceptions about its origins. In this case, if we look at the Ancient Egyptians as Asiatic peoples we would treat them and their culture in one way. If we see them as Africans we not only see them in a different light but we also must ascribe Africa with a glorious legacy that matches any other culture in human history. We would also look at the culture and philosophies of the Ancient Egyptians as having African insights instead of Asiatic ones. Those insights inform our knowledge bout other African traditions and we can also begin to understand in a deeper way the effect of Ancient Egyptian culture on African culture and also on the Asiatic as well. When we discover the deeper and more ancient practice of the postures system in Ancient Egypt that was called "Hatha Yoga" in India, we are able to find a new and expanded understanding of the practice that constitutes a discipline of spiritual practice that informs and revitalizes the Indian practices as well as all spiritual disciplines. $19.99 ISBN 1-884564-60-7

39. The Black Ancient Egyptians

175

This present volume, The Black Ancient Egyptians: The Black African Ancestry of the Ancient Egyptians, formed one subject in the larger work: The African Origins of Civilization, Religion, Yoga Mysticism and Ethics Philosophy. It was felt that this subject needed to be discussed because even in the early 21st century, the idea persists that the Ancient Egyptians were peoples originally from Asia Minor who came into North-East Africa. Yet there is ample evidence from ancient writings and perhaps more importantly, iconographical evidences from the Ancient Egyptians themselves that proves otherwise. This handy volume has been designed to be accessible to young adults and all others who would like to have an easy reference with documentation on this important subject. This is an important subject because the frame of reference with which we look at a culture depends strongly on our conceptions about its origins. in this case, if we look at the Ancient Egyptians as Asiatic peoples we would treat them and their culture in one way. If we see them as Africans we not only see them in a different light but we also must ascribe Africa with a glorious legacy that matches any other culture in human history. We would also look at the culture and philosophies of the Ancient Egyptians as having African insights instead of Asiatic ones. Those insights inform our knowledge bout other African traditions and we can also begin to understand in a deeper way the effect of Ancient Egyptian culture on African culture and also on the Asiatic as well. ISBN 1-884564-21-6 $19.99

40. The Limits of Faith: The Failure of Faith-based Religions and the Solution to the Meaning of Life

Is faith belief in something without proof? And if so is there never to be any proof or discovery? If so what is the need of intellect? If faith is trust in something that is real is that reality historical, literal or metaphorical or philosophical? If knowledge is an essential element in faith why should there by so much emphasis on believing and not on understanding in the modern practice of religion? This volume is a compilation of essays related to the nature of religious faith in the context of its inception in human history as well as its meaning for religious practice and relations between religions in modern times. Faith has come to be regarded as a virtuous goal in life. However, many people have asked how can it be that an endeavor that is supposed to be dedicated to spiritual upliftment has led to more conflict in human history than any other social factor? ISBN 1884564631 SOFT COVER - $19.99, ISBN 1884564623 HARD COVER -$28.95

41. Redemption of The Criminal Heart Through Kemetic Spirituality and Maat Philosophy

Special book dedicated to inmates, their families and members of the Law Enforcement community. ISBN: 1-884564-70-4 $5.00

42. COMPARATIVE MYTHOLOGY

What are Myth and Culture and what is their importance for understanding the development of societies, human evolution and the search for meaning? What is the purpose of culture and how do cultures evolve? What are the elements of a culture and how can those elements be broken down and the constituent parts of a culture understood and compared? How do cultures interact? How does enculturation occur and how do people interact with other cultures? How do the processes of acculturation and cooptation occur and what does this mean for the development of a society? How can the study of myths and the elements of culture help in understanding the meaning of life and the means to promote understanding and peace in the world of human activity? This volume is the exposition of a method for studying and comparing cultures, myths and other social aspects of a society. It is an expansion on the Cultural Category Factor Correlation method for studying and comparing myths, cultures, religions and other aspects of human culture. It was originally introduced in the year 2002. This volume contains an expanded treatment as well as several refinements along with examples of the application of the method. the apparent. I hope you enjoy these art renditions as serene reflections of the mysteries of life. ISBN: 1-884564-72-0

Book price $21.95

43. CONVERSATION WITH GOD: Revelations of the Important Questions of Life

$24.99 U.S.

This volume contains a grouping of some of the questions that have been submitted to Sebai Dr. Muata Ashby. They are efforts by many aspirants to better understand and practice the teachings of mystical spirituality. It is said that when sages are asked spiritual questions they are relaying the wisdom of God, the Goddess, the Higher Self, etc. There is a very special quality about the Q & A process that does not occur during a regular lecture session. Certain points come out that would not come out otherwise due to the nature of the process which ideally occurs after a lecture. Having been to a certain degree enlightened by a lecture certain new questions arise and the answers to these have the effect of elevating the teaching of the lecture to even higher levels. Therefore, enjoy these exchanges and may they lead you to enlightenment, peace and prosperity. Available Late Summer 2007 ISBN: 1-884564-68-2

44. MYSTIC ART PAINTINGS

(with Full Color images) This book contains a collection of the small number of paintings that I have created over the years. Some were used as early book covers and others were done simply to express certain spiritual feelings; some were created for no purpose except to express the joy of color and the feeling of relaxed freedom. All are to elicit mystical awakening in the viewer. Writing a book on philosophy is like sculpture, the more the work is rewritten the reflections and ideas become honed and take form and become clearer and imbued with intellectual beauty. Mystic music is like meditation, a world of its own that exists about 1 inch above ground wherein the musician does not touch the ground. Mystic Graphic Art is meditation in form, color, image and reflected image which opens the door to the reality behind the apparent. I hope you enjoy these art renditions and my reflections on them as serene reflections of the mysteries of life, as visual renditions of the philosophy I have written about over the years. ISBN 1-884564-69-0 $19.95

45. ANCIENT EGYPTIAN HIEROGLYPHS FOR BEGINNERS

This brief guide was prepared for those inquiring about how to enter into Hieroglyphic studies on their own at home or in study groups. First of all you should know that there are a few institutions around the world which teach how to read the Hieroglyphic text but due to the nature of the study there are perhaps only a handful of people who can read fluently. It is possible for anyone with average intelligence to achieve a high level of proficiency in reading inscriptions on temples and artifacts; however, reading extensive texts is another issue entirely. However, this introduction will give you entry into those texts if assisted by dictionaries and other aids. Most Egyptologists have a basic knowledge and keep dictionaries and notes handy when it comes to dealing with more difficult texts. Medtu Neter or the Ancient Egyptian hieroglyphic language has been considered as a "Dead Language." However, dead languages have always been studied by individuals who for the most part have taught themselves through various means. This book will discuss those means and how to use them most efficiently. ISBN 1884564429 **$28.95**

46. ON THE MYSTERIES: Wisdom of An Ancient Egyptian Sage -with Foreword by Muata Ashby
This volume, On the Mysteries, by Iamblichus (Abamun) is a unique form or scripture out of the Ancient Egyptian religious tradition. It is written in a form that is not usual or which is not usually found in the remnants of Ancient Egyptian scriptures. It is in the form of teacher and disciple, much like the Eastern scriptures such as Bhagavad Gita or the Upanishads. This form of writing may not have been necessary in Ancient times, because the format of teaching in Egypt was different prior to the conquest period by the Persians, Assyrians, Greeks and later the Romans. The question and answer format can be found but such extensive discourses and corrections of misunderstandings within the context of a teacher - disciple relationship is not usual. It therefore provides extensive insights into the times when it was written and the state of practice of Ancient Egyptian and other mystery religions. This has important implications for our times because we are today, as in the Greco-Roman period, also besieged with varied religions and new age philosophies as well as social strife and

war. How can we understand our times and also make sense of the forest of spiritual traditions? How can we cut through the cacophony of religious fanaticism, and ignorance as well as misconceptions about the mysteries on the other in order to discover the true purpose of religion and the secret teachings that open up the mysteries of life and the way to enlightenment and immortality? This book, which comes to us from so long ago, offers us transcendental wisdom that applied to the world two thousand years ago as well as our world today. ISBN 1-884564-64-X $25.95

47. The Ancient Egyptian Wisdom Texts -Compiled by Muata Ashby

The Ancient Egyptian Wisdom Texts are a genre of writings from the ancient culture that have survived to the present and provide a vibrant record of the practice of spiritual evolution otherwise known as religion or yoga philosophy in Ancient Egypt. The principle focus of the Wisdom Texts is the cultivation of understanding, peace, harmony, selfless service, self-control, Inner fulfillment and spiritual realization. When these factors are cultivated in human life, the virtuous qualities in a human being begin to manifest and sinfulness, ignorance and negativity diminish until a person is able to enter into higher consciousness, the coveted goal of all civilizations. It is this virtuous mode of life which opens the door to self-discovery and spiritual enlightenment. Therefore, the Wisdom Texts are important scriptures on the subject of human nature, spiritual psychology and mystical philosophy. The teachings presented in the Wisdom Texts form the foundation of religion as well as the guidelines for conducting the affairs of every area of social interaction including commerce, education, the army, marriage, and especially the legal system. These texts were sources for the famous 42 Precepts of Maat of the Pert M Heru (Book of the Dead), essential regulations of good conduct to develop virtue and purity in order to attain higher consciousness and immortality after death. ISBN1-884564-65-8 $18.95

48. THE KEMETIC TREE OF LIFE

THE KEMETIC TREE OF LIFE: Newly Revealed Ancient Egyptian Cosmology and Metaphysics for Higher Consciousness The Tree of Life is a roadmap of a journey which explains how Creation came into being and how it will end. It also explains what Creation is composed of and also what human beings are and what they are composed of. It also explains the process of Creation, how Creation develops, as well as who created Creation and where that entity may be found. It also explains how a human being may discover that entity and in so doing also discover the secrets of Creation, the meaning of life and the means to break free from the pathetic condition of human limitation and mortality in order to discover the higher realms of being by discovering the principles, the levels of existence that are beyond the simple physical and material aspects of life. This book contains color plates   **ISBN: 1-884564-74-7**

$27.95 U.S.

49-MATRIX OF AFRICAN PROVERBS: The Ethical and Spiritual Blueprint
This volume sets forth the fundamental principles of African ethics and their practical applications for use by individuals and organizations seeking to model their ethical policies using the Traditional African values and concepts of ethical human behavior for the proper sustenance and management of society. Furthermore, this book will provide guidance as to how the Traditional African Ethics may be viewed and applied, taking into consideration the technological and social advancements in the present. This volume also presents the principles of ethical culture, and references for each to specific injunctions from Traditional African Proverbial Wisdom Teachings. These teachings are compiled from varied Pre-colonial African societies including Yoruba, Ashanti, Kemet, Malawi, Nigeria, Ethiopia, Galla, Ghana and many more. ISBN 1-884564-77-1

50- Growing Beyond Hate: Keys to Freedom from Discord, Racism, Sexism, Political Conflict, Class Warfare, Violence, and How to Achieve Peace and Enlightenment---

INTRODUCTION: WHY DO WE HATE? Hatred is one of the fundamental motivating aspects of human life; the other is desire. Desire can be of a worldly nature or of a spiritual, elevating nature. Worldly desire and hatred are like two sides of the same coin in that human life is usually swaying from one to the other; but the question is why? And is there a way to satisfy the desiring or hating mind in such a way as to find peace in life? Why do human beings go to war? Why do human beings perpetrate violence against one another? And is there a way not just to understand the phenomena but to resolve the issues that plague humanity and could lead to a more harmonious society? Hatred is perhaps the greatest scourge of humanity in that it leads to misunderstanding, conflict and untold miseries of life and clashes between individuals, societies and nations. Therefore, the riddle of Hatred, that is, understanding the sources of it and how to confront, reduce and even eradicate it so as to bring forth the fulfillment in life and peace for society, should be a top priority for social scientists, spiritualists and philosophers. This book is written from the perspective of spiritual philosophy based on the mystical wisdom and sema or yoga philosophy of the Ancient Egyptians. This philosophy, originated and based in the wisdom of Shetaut Neter, the Egyptian Mysteries, and Maat, ethical way of life in society and in spirit, contains Sema-Yogic wisdom and understanding of lifes predicaments that can allow a human being of any ethnic group to understand and overcome the causes of hatred, racism, sexism, violence and disharmony in life, that plague human society. ISBN: 1-884564-81-X

Ancient Egyptian Economics

Order Form

Telephone orders: Call Toll Free: 1(305) 378-6253. Have your AMEX, Optima, Visa or MasterCard ready.

Fax orders: 1-(305) 378-6253   E-MAIL ADDRESS: Semayoga@aol.com

Postal Orders: Sema Institute of Yoga, P.O. Box 570459, Miami, Fl. 33257. USA.

Please send the following books and / or tapes.

ITEM

_____Cost \$_____

_____Cost \$_____

_____Cost \$_____

_____Cost \$_____

Total \$_____

Name:_____

Physical
Address:_____

City:_____ State:_____ Zip:_____

Sales tax: Please add 6.5% for books shipped to Florida addresses

_____Shipping: \$6.50 for first book and .50¢ for each additional

_____Payment:_____

_____Check -Include Driver License #:

_____

_____Credit card: _____ Visa, _____ MasterCard, _____ Optima,_____ AMEX.

Card number:_____

Name on card:_____ Exp. date:_____/_____

www.ingramcontent.com/pod-product-compliance
Lightning Source LLC
Chambersburg PA
CBHW072133020426
42334CB00018B/1778